Soul Ingredients:

Creating life's potential today

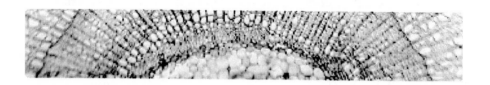

PAGONA, HHC, M.Ac., GAPS™

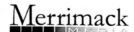

Library of Congress Cataloging-in-Publication Data
Pagona HHC, M. Ac, GAPS™
Soul Ingredients: Creating life's potential today
Includes bibliographical references and index.
ISBN 978-1-939166-17
1. Healing   2. Nutrition   3. Self- help   4. Title

Cover design: Tal Kelly of www.talkelly.com
Hair: Maité Lopez Ramirez of www.bradleyanddiegel.com
Photography: Mack Dillingham of www.dillinghammedia.com

A Merrimack Media edition

17 January 2014

Dear Erin,

ALLOW YOURSELF A NEW PERSPECTIVE.

EMBRACE A NEW EXPERIENCE.

BE OPEN TO LIFE,

LOVE & MANIFESTING YOUR GREATNESS.

INSPIRE OTHERS TO LIVE THEIRS.

May you always
be happy, expansive,
sweet & live life on
Purpose.
So happy you're in my life...
Thank you for the joy that is you...

Payne

SOUL

Menu A: Concepts & related ingredients

Menu B: Food & related ingredients

INGREDIENTS

Menu C: Healing Modalities

SOUL INGREDIENTS

ACKNOWLEDGMENTS

I t is an honor to share this book globally and it would not have been possible without my parents, who are role models. Μαμα και μπαμπα, χιλια εφχαριστο για την αγαπη και ηπομονει σας. You embody love, hard work and perseverance and for this I am grateful.

Sue and Aaron Singleton, I sit in gratitude for your compassionate healing and wisdom. Over a decade ago, you propelled me into knowing thyself and listened patiently as I looked outside for answers, gently nudging me to look inward.

To the men I dated, you helped me 'see' the real me and were instrumental in my soul learning lessons. Thanks for the 'ugly' and wondrous moments.

To my sisters, Γεωργια, Πασχαλια and Ολγα, how honored I am to be an aunt to your precious children and a witness to your unfoldment. All we experienced as Greek Americans in the U.S. brought us to a greater understanding, respect and love for sisterhood. Thank you for making me laugh and inspiring me to greater heights.

To my nieces Eleni, Alexandra, Sofia and my nephews Dimitri, Tolie, David Jr. and Gianni, your souls leave a never ending smile on my heart. You enrich my life and I give thanks for the treasure of being your Aunt.

I love you- Γιαγια Παγωνα, Παπου Πασχαλι, Παπου Δημητρι and Γιαγια Ολγα. To me you embody wisdom and knowing from my ancestors. Although you passed on, your blood is part of my blood, your wisdom in the brain cells of my cranium. How blessed I am to have frolicked in Greece and America moments with you...

To friends: Agata, Alexa, Andy, Christine, Dorota, Errol, Jonathan, Melinda, Monica, Rafa, Taly and Tanya, thanks for your lifeline of love, humor and support. Without your light rays, my world would be dimmer. Taly, I am honored to showcase your talent on the beautiful cover!

To my MM group, you understand, embrace and love me for me. Thank you for the journey into the Mind with Bob Proctor and friends.

To Bob Proctor, your 13 month coaching program was the vehicle to unleash my quantum leap. Mary Morrissey, Peggy McColl and Gay Hendricks, you are magnetic forces of abundance radiating beautifully in my life. Thank you for your gifts to humanity.

To Joshua Rosenthal, for creating a school and community of health coaches who globally empower humanity. Thanks for the truth of Integrative Nutrition.

To Lenedra J. Carroll, thank you for embracing me in your home; the gift of your book *The Architecture of All Abundance* and your gentle words of wisdom. You embody peace, compassion and strength and for this I am eternally grateful.

I remain blessed for my years of culinary and catering experience and food exploration. Thank you to the Chefs, Pastry Chefs and everyone I am blessed to call culinary friends and wizards! Delicious and nutritious food fuels my soul!

To Del Blank, a big hug and thank you for embracing me into your medical world and for the gift of working with you and many talented nurses, doctors and medical staff in the ER. Those years and memories are forever etched in my brain, as is every patient encounter.

A huge thank you to Dennis Vanasse, for the opportunity to serve college students and learn from them. Appreciation and gratitude to Lisa Leblanc, PhD and Lisa Driscoll, PhD for the honor of adjunct faculty teaching World Cultures.

To Jenny Hudson, CEO of Merrimack Media, thank you for embracing me and this book into your family. You and your team are publishing gems! To Colin Miller, thank you for your talent creating beautiful online websites.

To the magnificent Spirit; creator(s); multidimensional realities and the etheric realm of possibilities, I am grateful for your presence. Ten years ago you were an invisible seed in my question, unasked. You are real and I embrace you.

To the souls who crossed my path on my travels, young and old, frail and strong, thank you for blessing me, for even a fleeting moment with your beauty. You brought infinite Awareness to these once sheltered eyes.

PAGONA

To the curanderas; herbologists; midwives; Shamans and all traditional healers of the world, thank you for sharing your path of healing and ancient wisdom. I sit humbled and at your service. Planetary consciousness is vibrating higher because of your gifts.

To the continents of Africa; Asia; Europe; North America and South America and the 28 countries my soul was blessed to witness, I thank you for your wisdom, food, people and ways of being. We are all one in this magnificent space called Gaia. Thanks for increasing my awareness and allowing my physical temple to be a vehicle spreading unity, Oneness and healing. Every adventure transformed me and continually infuses my consciousness.

A special thanks to all contributors- both personal and whose books and words grace these pages. You are a gift to humanity. Thanks for allowing a glimpse into your life and gifting the world your words. To every author and philosophy I was and continually am blessed to encounter, thanks for your gift of wisdom.

Thank you to all who purchase and read the words on this paper. Without open minded, eager and progressive humans, this book would remain a dormant, unsprouted idea...

Χιλια εφχαριστο. Χιλια εφχαριστο. Χιλια εφχαριστο.

SOUL INGREDIENTS

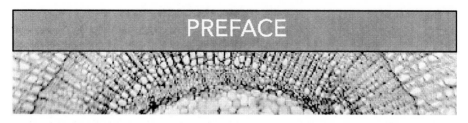

PREFACE

WHY BRING SOUL INGREDIENTS INTO EXISTENCE?

"To know that you don't know is the beginning of knowing."
Confucius

Awareness, happiness, health, living on purpose and embracing one's potential seem happily married to some while divorced from others. They are objective and subjective simultaneously. At times, it surprises some and shocks others, as to how aware and empowered or unaware and disempowered, humanity appears to be. As one of my mentors, Bob Proctor states: "There is only 1 problem in the world that anyone will ever have and that is ignorance."

With peace, gratitude, self -empowerment, higher consciousness and attuned living come love; life; laughter; forgiveness; compassion; empathy; humor; kindness; peace; generosity and everything known and unknown to humanity. How can one do what one is unaware of (on all levels- including intuition and multidimensional realities)? Yes awareness exists on more than the physical plane, 3D dimension and reality 'you' call Earth with the reality 'you' say is yours...

Before studying energy in the form of Traditional Chinese Medicine (TCM) and the esoteric philosophies of the world, my awareness of the metaphysical, the unseen, the etheric was limited. Now, daily, I embrace each activity and person and act on the energy present. Awareness of the food and thoughts that nourish me generates tremendous joy rippling throughout my physical temple, spirit body and soul body.

We are part of a grander Universe than that which our physical eyes perceive; something so magnificent that the human mind, in its current state of allowing, may not comprehend. We belong to a magical energetic 'space' that humanity, Gaia and the cosmic consciousness ask us to embrace daily. The question, dear reader, is what choices do you choose? How do these decisions manifest in your life? Are you ready to embrace another option? Are you ready for a thought provoking journey into your power, healing and your mind?

The experience of being the oldest of 4 Greek American daughters brought an interesting mix of Greek tradition, assimilation and anomaly to my young eyes. Part of the integration involved transcending my negative thought patterns. For many years, the ingredients in my life were toxic. Worry impregnated my mind and manifested in a myriad of unsuspecting clues. The first was an uncertainty and inability to make decisions. Understanding outside my paradigm was like speaking a foreign language. Worry and its friends were debilitating enemies, making large contributions to emotional uneasiness and toxicity and the manifestation of an 11 lb. benign mass (it looked as if I was 7 months pregnant) in my abdomen.

Once the mass was removed, I was different. Life was gloriously full and abundant. Peace, trust and happiness flowed easily. It was as if I gave birth to a new world, the outer environment mirroring my inner sanctuary. Worry was no longer a welcomed guest at my table. It is foreign to me now and difficult to imagine who that 'other' person was.

Subconsciously, an inner stirring occurred one day that propelled me to this book. I was seeking a compact book encompassing global healing modalities, science, spirituality, nutrition and more and was unable to locate it. Hence my journey began. The journey took 10 + years and birthed this book. It is by no means comprehensive as that would house infinite volumes yet it encompasses many disciplines and explores research, concepts and insights. May this Greek American's humble endeavor to the world attune you, your senses and your 'mind'; question your perception of who 'you' are and empower you with knowledge to make healthy, informed decisions. While some may agree with concepts presented, others may disagree. I embrace and encourage all perspectives as long as one thinks.

Many ask "Why are you so happy?" A smile permeates my face as I respond it is housed in you. While this stifles many, others understand. It is awareness of the human condition and humanity's suffering and programming while 'unlearning' paradigms, which fuels my happiness. Much of my knowledge and paradigms were taught to me in a manner that disempowered me. Until I allowed 'truth' to steep into the inner recesses of my DNA and took responsibility for my awareness, for my life and thoughts and actions; no knowledge could act for me. True power hails from within and like Gandhi said, "You can chain me, you can torture me, you can even destroy this body but you will never imprison my mind."

For those desiring greater health, empowerment and awareness, may I extend an invitation to embrace this book with an open mind while maintaining a deep appreciation for all aspects of your life. Witnessing raw poverty in Ethiopia and encountering limbless children in Cambodia (land mines are still prevalent) put me in an altered space. When the Cambodian tour guide mentioned former Khmer Rouge child soldiers in the streets are met with love and forgiveness; my soul rethought healing, spirituality, food and the ingredients in my life.

For the gift of travel to 28 countries, no words can describe its profound impact on my cells. As Thich Nhat Hanh stated, "It is difficult to explain to children in the "overdeveloped" nations that not all children in the world have such beautiful and nourishing food. Awareness of this fact alone can help us overcome many of our own psychological pains."

Gratitude is embedded in the life force and I sit, grateful for all blessings and opportunities, at times cleverly disguised as 'obstacles' or circumstances that 'appear' to not serve my highest good. How blessed to be born to Greek immigrants who instilled in me the importance of traditions; family; honesty, respect; knowledge and work ethic. My parents arrived in America with little, not knowing a word of English, yet are grand to me.

We are all one. We are different faces, different races yet all spiritual beings living in a physical body, all cells responding to our innermost thoughts and beliefs. Thanks to Bob Proctor, for W.A.I.T: What Am I Thinking? Ask yourself this question when you feel negativity manifesting as unworthiness, guilt, lack, etc. Now visualize and think of the most beautiful baby you know. How does that feel? Congratulations- you just experienced the power of thought...

Soul Ingredients is meant as suggestions, not rules for life. It is not a comprehensive list and is purposely written as such. Some vignettes are longer while others are short. This is exactly as it should be. It is meant as mind stimulation so that you look deeper into aspects you are attracted to.

The Invitation to expand in selected sections is intended as suggestions to open a greater awareness door in your life. Use it or choose not to. Peruse the concepts, healing modalities, ways of thinking with an open mind, embracing what resonates with YOU... May it enhance your soul, incorporating ingredients of your choice. Enjoy mixing, playing and digesting each!

May this endeavor serve and empower you to find your inner constant smile. As Einstein stated, "The important thing is not to stop questioning."

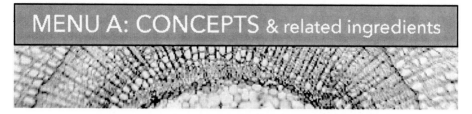

ABUNDANCE SURROUNDS YOU

"Creating abundance [is] not about creating a life of luxury for everybody on this planet; it's about creating a life of possibility."
Peter Diamandis

What is abundance? According to psychic Hans Christian King, "Abundance sits on your heart that you are already enough. If you are already abundant, abundance finds you." Abundance is a state of understanding that we are enough and have everything we need to exist. When one understands the truth, one embraces the abundance of the world. If you live in lack in your mind, this 'belief' becomes your reality. Like many of you, I was unaware of this life changing thought until I studied with Bob Proctor. Wayne Dyer reminds you that "Doing what you love is the cornerstone of having abundance in your life."

Growing up in a household of strict Greek immigrant parents presented challenges and growth opportunities. My non Greek friends attended the usual events- Girl Scouts; dates; the prom, etc. For me, life involved school; homework; working on weekends; cleaning the house Saturdays and enjoying mom's homemade food. Burgers, pizza and sandwiches were a treat. I remember fighting to attend the Junior prom and after an hour intensely debating why I was going to go and mentioning my Greek friend was attending, my wish was granted.

The environment was simple, sharing the top bunk bed in a room with my sister, housed in a three decker. Abundance was not part of my lenses. My sisters and I learned to buy only what was needed.

Today I sit in gratitude with love and appreciation for my upbringing. During my teenage years, gratitude was foreign to me. Gratitude was replaced by anger and frustration. These feelings were 'fed' by sugar, leading to a dependence that created an 11 lb. abdominal mass. Yes- sugar, emotions such as anger, resentment and worry have physical affects in the body. Devote a minute of your life digesting that. For me, these, entangled with my repetitive negative 'stories', helped create such toxicity that a mass the size of a 7 month pregnancy manifested in my physical temple.

My parents, like many immigrants, did their best with their knowledge. No training manuals existed on how to live as a Greek in America. Daily attempts at assimilation were their coursework. Homework reflected what worked and didn't in their sparse spare time. Dad worked two jobs and Sunday was his one day off- our cherished family day.

Although my upbringing didn't present me with opportunities to bask in abundance, my travels and catering experiences did. Cooking in million dollar homes, surrounding myself with opulence demonstrated anything is possible. Traveling to beautiful destinations, witnessing the poor and richly abundant areas showed me life's polarity. For poverty to exist, another reality- wealth must also exist. Just as day turns into night, 'poor' people can become wealthy. In fact, Bob Proctor shares this in *You Were Born Rich!* You are all born rich. Abundance is a state of mind you are born with.

Invitation to expand:
Abundance surrounds you. Where can you place yourself to 'see' this? What is your 'story' about abundance? Where you also raised in a similar manner that limited what you thought possible? Did your reality allow expansive possibilities? If not, who do you know with a different reality willing to entertain you? Listen to his/her story and feel what is possible. In the child's mind, everything is possible. It is also in your life. Choose to embrace what is yours- abundance.

"ALLOW THE YOU TO COME OUT"

Rev. Michael B. Beckwith

"Acceptance is not submission; it is an acknowledgement of the facts of the situation. It helps decide your future course of action. Those who accept things that cannot be changed are as

wise as grass that grows in the riverbeds. Those who refuse to accept are like trees. When a storm blows, the grass accepts and survives but the tree falls to the power of the wind. Acceptance is an important character that we have to inculcate in us, to survive successfully in this world."

K C Thiesen

For years, I lived in a world of resisting the 'not so good' that entered my life. It appeared that acceptance and allowing were *xeno* (Greek for foreign) to me. My mind entertained everything except allowing and often knew only how to pretend to exert control on the situation.

This book was a lesson in allowing. Originally it was to be a joint venture which transformed into this with a 'fixed' deadline. However, whenever I thought it was done, the Universe unveiled another dimension, seminar, person or book be incorporated. Thus, my intuition led me to its completion, if I can say it is complete.

Control is an illusion and everything occurs as it should. Observe a flower blooming. Does it try to control its height? No. It grows, almost gracefully, given the proper nutrients, at exactly the time it will and for the length of time it will. Everything occurs in its own rhythm, swaying perfectly in unison to nature and its surroundings. Humans are like flowers. Given proper support, love, nutrients and knowledge, they bloom. Conversely, lack of love and nutrients yield the opposite.

In the film *Spiritual Liberation,* you are urged "Allow the you to come out." When I did, I embraced myself, in my wholeness and all I am blessed with. My eyes were no longer clouded with indecision and the inability to allow and accept.

Osho states "Accept yourself. Delight in your being! There is no need to hanker for any meaning. Moment to moment is full of meaning." Allow, accept and embrace you. As Michael Bernard Beckwith states in Agape Spiritual Center's mission statement, "(Realize) you are a unique emanation of God, the Love-Intelligence governing the Universe." Embrace your Divinity and beauty knowing that unconditional love is your birthright.

Part of allowing is trusting that everything occurs exactly as it should, at the perfect place and at the perfect time with the perfect people. When one accepts that one is the creator of his/her life and takes responsibility, one's life changes and transcends to a higher frequency.

ACKNOWLEDGEMENT

"Acknowledgment is embracing what serves and that which can be let go. In essence, it drives clarity and action for without either, one remains stuck."
Pagona

Andrew Stanton once shared "A major threshold is passed when you mature enough to acknowledge what drives you and to take the wheel and steer it." When you acknowledge and therefore accept the condition of your life, you embrace all possibilities. No longer are you the victim but the possibilitarian. Acknowledging enables you to accept responsibility for your life, full responsibility and act accordingly.

Invitation to expand:
What is important for you to acknowledge? What is important for you to accept? What needs letting go of? What steps can you take NOW to do this?

ACTION

"It's the little things you do that can make a big difference. What are you attempting to accomplish? What little thing can you do today that will make you more effective? You are probably only one step away from greatness." Bob Proctor

When Henry David Thoreau performed his experiment of living in Walden Woods in Concord, MA, many insights came to him. One insight was "Go confidently in the direction of your dreams. Live the life you have imagined." Take action daily, towards what you wish to manifest. Mary Morrissey reminds you that "Everything comes out of thought. Act as if."

Ralph Waldo Emerson once said "What you do speaks so loudly that I cannot hear what you say." What if you did what you not only thought impossible but thrived instead of survived? Most people live in a survival mentality- working, eating, socializing to the extent they believe they can. Some walk their entire lives without knowing the possibility of a different action, reliving fixed beliefs, or paradigms of their mind on a new day, in a new place, yet the actions remain unchanged. Many put off what they can do because their illusion of fear is greater than their desire for change. Og Mandino reiterated the importance of action against inaction by stating "Action will destroy your procrastination."

Zig Ziglar spoke about many topics including selling, influencing others and taking action. He stated, "The major difference between the big shot and the little shot is the big shot is just a little shot who kept on shooting." Attitude and perseverance are critical components with action. Aristotle once said "You are what you repeatedly do. Excellence is not an event - it is a habit."

T. Harv Eker, in his book, *The Secrets of a Millionaire Mind,* reminds you that T→ F →A→ R. Thoughts (T) lead to feelings (F) which lead to action (A) which leads to results (R). These are discussed further in the FEELINGS and THOUGHTS sections. George S. Patton stated "Never tell people HOW to do things. Tell them what to do and they will surprise you with their ingenuity."

In *Conversations with God, Book II,* Neale Donald Walsch shares "A life lived by choice is a life of conscious action. A life lived by chance is a life of unconscious reaction." When you re-act, you relive an action you took part in before. Take creative action based on your soul's wisdom and not that of your mind because as Walsch states "The soul creates and the mind reacts."

Invitation to expand:
How can you know you are succeeding? Review what you do daily, your habits and ask yourself, do these serve your dream or your procrastination? Is this action moving you closer to your goal or is it allowing you to stay comfortable? As Aristotle once said "One must learn by doing the thing, for though you think you know it, you have no certainty until you try."

AFFIRMATIONS/DECLARATIONS

Below you'll find affirmations/declarations to incorporate into your daily life. These are most effective with action, faith, gratefulness and a strong intention to improve your life.

T. Harv Eker, president of Peak Potentials Training, suggests using **VAKS** (Visual, Auditory, Kinesthetic and Spirit) techniques to integrate your left and right brain while repeating affirmations. For Visual, clasp hands in front of you and move hands from left to right forming a figure 8 while your eyes follow your thumbs (do not move your head). For Auditory, massage the rim of both ears simultaneously, starting at the top of ears. Repeat for 30 seconds while saying affirmation. For Kinesthetic, stand with arms raised and bend elbows. Raise left leg and twist body to touch your right elbow. Repeat with right leg. Do this while repeating affirmation for 30 seconds. For Spirit, place both hands over your heart, close your eyes and repeat affirmation for 30 seconds.

"I am a child of the infinite; I have a right and responsibility for more abundance in my life." Mary Morrissey

"I AM AT ONE WITH THE ABUNDANCE OF THE UNIVERSE." Rev. Michael Bernard Beckwith

"I am so happy and grateful now that _____." Bob Proctor (fill in the blank with present tense goal/desire, target date, etc.) Ex- I am so happy and grateful now that money comes to me continuously, etc.

"I am a money magnet. Thank you, thank you, thank you." Peak Potentials Training (Repeat this with great belief and enthusiasm)

"I willingly release the thoughts and things that clutter my mind. I release (fill in person's name) to their highest good."

"I easily clear out the excess clutter in my home, body and mind." Julie Dittmar, Hypnotherapy for Peak Potentials Training

"I take responsibility for my life." Julie Dittmar, Hypnotherapy for Peak Potentials Training

"I have immense courage and take action." Julie Dittmar, Hypnotherapy for Peak Potentials Training

"Each day, in every way, I make wise, healthy choices." Julie Dittmar, Hypnotherapy for Peak Potentials Training

"I acknowledge, appreciate and respect my body." Julie Dittmar, Hypnotherapy for Peak Potentials Training

"I go with the flow and succeed with ease." Julie Dittmar for Peak Potentials Training

"I commit to being lucky now and forever." Gay Hendricks, Ph.D.

Co-founder of www.phoenixhealingcenter; author; healer and the late educator Dr. Sidney Wolf, shared this mantra in Sedona in June 2012: "I GIVE MY BODY, MIND & SOUL PERMISSION TO HEAL & BE IN BALANCE." Tap both hemispheres of cerebral cortex- tapping top of head and heart. The heart has an electromagnetic field 50 times larger than the brain. You are supercharging this field when you do this.

Gay Hendricks, Ph.D. offers a powerful Ultimate Success Mantra (USM). He suggests saying this a few times in your mind and allowing it to resonate. "I expand in abundance, success and love every day as I inspire those around me to do the same."

Invitation to expand:

In addition to the above affirmations, you may also use the following affirmation related to the power of Mind I learned in a 13 month coaching program with Bob Proctor. Although it is longer than others, it may resonate with you.

"My mind is my center of Divine Operation. Divine Operation is already for expansion and expression and production of something beyond what went before, something new; not included in past experience, though proceeding out of it by an orderly sequence of growth. Therefore, since the Divine can't change its inherent nature, it must operate in the same manner in me, in my special world of which I am the center. It will move forward to produce new conditions, always in advance of any that have gone before."
Thomas Troward

ALIVENESS

"Don't worry about what the world needs. Ask yourself what makes you come alive and do that. What the world needs is people who have come alive."
Dr. Howard Thurman

What is aliveness? Daphne Rose Kingma gives a beautiful description with these words "Aliveness is energy. It's the juice, the vitality, and the passion that wakes up our cells every morning. It's what makes us want to dance. It's the energy that moves a relationship from the status quo to something grander and more expansive, something that makes our hearts beat faster, our minds and our eyes open wider than ever before. Everything is of interest to a person who is truly alive, whether it's a challenge, a loving moment, a bucket of grief, or a glimpse of beauty."

Invitation to expand:
What makes you come alive? How often do you do this? How can you incorporate more of that into your life?

ANCHOR INTO YOUR TRUE SELF

"Begin to consciously break your agreement with the mediocrity present in the tyranny of trends."
Taken from the film *Spiritual Liberation.*

What does it mean to anchor into your true self? Do you recognize you have a true self? If so, what is it? Your true self, or Divine self is that soul that is in touch with the infinite, with spirit, with Divinity. Take all labels away and see it for what it is- a higher consciousness within you. It does not judge, label, ridicule but comes from a place of love, compassion and guidance.

How do you anchor into your true self? It involves accessing the collective mind while releasing the mediocre, in all ways. It involves introspection, faith in the unseen and daily devotion to the powerful creator within. It entails being and living in your unique spirit; in the physical temple you were blessed with; embracing the gifts and talents bestowed upon you.

Psychiatrist and New York Times bestseller, Judith Orloff, MD states "We must first reprogram ourselves by envisioning the extent of our vastness and challenge anyone who insists on making us small." Often, you play small, in a relationship, your career, or other parts of your life while not fully grasping what you do. I like to say "If you knew how brilliant you are, it would astound you and your playing small would die forever."

When you embrace the power within you and like Dr. Orloff states challenge those who attempt to make you small, you tell the Universe you know who you are and you choose not to allow others to disempower you. The mediocre may not understand you, yet you continue to follow the light within, allowing yours to shine brightly like the sun's luminosity. In the words of Albert Einstein "Great spirits have always encountered violent opposition from mediocre minds." Be great and live in your true, authentic self.

My true self may be odd, different, unusual than most yet it is mine. It is what I bless and embrace and was placed on this planet to be. In a world of separation and illusion, it comforts me like a hot cup of hot chocolate sweetened with raw honey during a snowstorm. Being labeled 'crazy' is now embraced where it once was not. I meet it with a smile and offer blessings to the person who utters it. My nephew Tolie once called me "Odd" to which I replied "Are you sure I'm not even?" He lips curled up unfolding a beautiful smile.

ASK FOR YOUR DESIRES/ASK BETTER, BIGGER QUESTIONS

In Feb 2010, while on a conference call with Mary Morrissey, I asked about keeping your mind on your vision when you have pressure. Mary's response was brilliant: "Ask bigger questions. If you ask struggle questions, you attract struggle." As a lifelong inquisitive student, many who know me know I ask millions of questions. I learned to craft my questions wisely and think about what is most conducive to my day's lesson. Also, why am I asking this question when a better question may be asked? Remember, the quality of your questions determines the quality of your answers. Ask wisely.

Invitation to expand:
Pay attention to the questions you ask. What questions do you ask yourself and others? What questions are you asking the Universe? Are you playing small and safe or are you asking expanding questions? What do you expect? Are you expecting great results? Why didn't you ask for these things in the past? Did you expect them?

Ask for what you desire. Part of asking questions is listening to the reponse and taking action. You may believe you will not receive your desire and therefore do not ask. Change that. Expect what you need; anticipate it like you anticipate the birth of your newborn child. It is as simple as asking for what you desire; taking steps to manifest it and asserting perseverance and compassionate determination during your journey. Ask for what you need and it will be provided. It may not be today or tomorrow yet it will occur if you believe, ask and persist. Ask, expect great things to manifest and take action.

YOUR GREATEST ASSET-ATTITUDE

"The greatest discovery of my generation is that human beings can alter their lives by altering their attitudes of mind."
William James

The following quote on my wall, I received in college. It is a beautiful example of the power of attitude. Charles R. Swindoll stated "The longer I live, the more I realize the impact of attitude on life. Attitude, to me, is more important than facts. It is more important than the past, education, money, circumstances, failure, successes, what other people think or say or do. It is more important than appearance, giftedness or skill. It will make or break a company...a church... a home. We have a choice everyday regarding the attitude we will embrace for that day. We cannot change our past...we cannot change the fact that people will act in a certain way. The only thing we can do is play on the one string we have and that is our attitude. I am convinced that life is 10% what happens to me and 90% of how I react to it. So it is with you... we are in charge of our Attitudes."

What is attitude? Bob Proctor gives a great definition by stating "Attitude is a composite of thoughts (conscious mind); feelings (subconscious mind) and actions which produce results." In other words, attitude = T (thoughts) + F (feelings) + A (actions). What you think about comes from what you know to be true. This determines your thoughts which lead to your feelings and ultimately your actions.

Shantidera, a great Indian Buddhist sage reminds you "If you can do something about a bad situation, why be angry about it? Just do it! If you can't do anything about it, why hurt yourself more by getting angry about it?

Remain cheerful and you stay free, no matter what happens, life or death."

Invitation to expand:
What attitudes do you hold? How do these attitudes make you feel? What actions result from these attitudes? Expect beautiful, remarkable and wonderful things to occur!! What you expect you may receive. Never think about what you do not want. A consistent change of attitude in a positive direction will change your life.

3 QUESTIONS:

The idea came to me in January 2012 to document what Awareness means to you. This lead to 2 further questions: **1) What does Happiness mean to you? 2) What does Health mean to you?** Many were honored to be included and I am grateful and humbled by their responses. How honored I am to partake in that process and for their wisdom that graces these pages. Thank you for saying yes to this endeavor and for sharing yourselves.

WHAT DOES AWARENESS MEAN TO YOU?

Jonathan C Cordeiro, Jccimagineer, Purist, Human
"Awareness is rooted in truth. If you are aware of the truths that are the fabrics of your individual make up, you will be more aware of your decisions, actions and surroundings.

I am often told I am a "purist". A purist in the sense that I am pure in my thoughts, actions, questions, beliefs and most importantly, the admittance of my wrongs and faults. I believe this is caused by my ability to be aware. Reality is based on an individual's perception. We see the world through our own individual lens which allows for many different interpretations of the same view. However, not everyone is able to process what they see or experience on a daily basis. We were born into this world with 5 senses and the ability to sense energy from all matter around us. As we refine these senses and master the ability to use them, we become more aware of ourselves and what makes up our surrounding energies."

Luis Alfonso Dau, PhD in International Business/Strategy:

"Awareness is the realization that we are here and now; that we are mortal yet eternal; that we are beings of light; that we are love and unconditionally loved, that we are intimately connected with everything and everyone; that we are but a single cell in the body of humanity and yet a full universe exists within each of us and that the only constant in life is change."

Deb DeLisi, artist, owner of www.delisiart.com:

"Awareness is applying consciousness to the present moment. What you are doing, feeling, thinking or being...wherever you are in that instant, experience it by applying consciousness to it. Look at everything as if you are the creator of it."

Gay Hendricks, PhD, relationship expert, author of 36 books:

"Awareness means several things to me. First, it's an action: the act of including something in your attention that was previously outside it. For example, you're in an argument and you suddenly become aware of the sensations of fear in your belly. Instead of continuing the angry exchanges, you talk about your fear and the argument ceases. There's also a deeper awareness, an always-on background of pure consciousness that I become aware of when I meditate. It seems to be behind all thoughts, kind of like a whiteboard with no writing on it. It has an oceanic vastness to it and is very comforting to experience." February 2012

Kahuna Kalei'iliahi:

"Awareness is a consciousness of the Human that is connected to not only their own Divinity but to the planet and all living things...the state of mind that sees no separation. This connection allows the Human to be alert to what is happening in and around themselves and other living things and behave appropriately to it. It allows the Human to have compassion and empathy, for their consciousness is undivided."

Pascalia Mattioli, artist, mother, sister to Pagona:

"Awareness means living in the moment, enjoying what is around you and realizing who you really are as a person. Awareness can lead to peacefulness, feeling connected to your honest self and then to the world, others, nature and most importantly, feeling God's presence. Awareness means being open-minded and taking charge of what you need, want and feel at that moment in time."

Peggy McColl, NY Times best-selling author:
"Awareness is like a staircase: each step brings you up one more level, and the farther you ascend, the more you can see."

Mary Morrissey, author, speaker, visionary empowerment specialist:
"Your awareness is your access to the infinite side of your nature where there is no limit to what you can see, do, be." 25 January 2012

Todd Ovokaitys, MD:
"Awareness is a core attribute of being. It is a requirement for sentience and the evolution of body, mind and being. With respect to the notion of holographic awareness, it is postulated that it is awareness itself that creates the wave form matrix that condenses from zero point energy the structure of the universe itself and its dynamics of flow.

While almost any other substance or attribute can be stretched to a level of excess, awareness is a rare factor that having more of is virtually always better. Awareness may be much more than that which allows the perception of existence; its presence and developing it in higher degrees may be the very purpose of existence."

Bob Proctor, author of *You Were Born Rich*, Chairman, Life Success Productions and Law Of Attraction living master:
"Awareness is seeing something with the eye of the one, with your mind that you couldn't see before. It's like when a baby is born, a baby is not aware of the difference between a male and a female. A baby has to become aware of the difference in gender. We have to become aware of how to do better than we are doing. We raise our consciousness and we see what we couldn't see before. Everything already is here. The way is here. Seek first the kingdom of expansion and all these things will be given to you. How? Because you become aware of their presence." 25 January 2012

Linda Roach, writer:

"The height of awareness is the realization that we are incredibly loved, supported and connected beings that can do anything we set our unlimited minds to."

David Roe, Master Mind friend:

"Awareness is the ability to recognize that the world is truly perfect because everything is balanced. It is the recognition of the balance that keeps you grounded, puts a stop to stress and worry and places a smile on your face even when a situation looks rather grim."

Sandra Roe, Master Mind friend:

"It means listening to my intuition and listening to my body. Noticing what I am thinking, how I am feeling and what I am saying. This creates my world. Awareness at the level of being as Deepak Chopra says in his meditation cd. Understanding that everything is connected. Letting go and being, knowing that I create my world."

Dr. Dave Smiley, Creator, *The Inner Weigh®*, A documentary film about Spirit, Mind and weight loss, http://TheInnerWeigh.com:

"Awareness,
Knowing I have all
        I need,
Breathing . . .
Breathing . . .
Breathing . . .
Giving thanks for all
        that is,
I am blessed."

Andrew Thom, CPA, CFP, CMA, MBA:

"Awareness is the ability to not only see the clouds but to see behind them."

Thaddeus III, Relaxationist/Creator of www.eyeamu2.com:
"Awareness is the recognition of your surroundings. When we are clear of distractions we will be able to hear our intuition and our inner voice. A great example is a deer in the woods carefully walking and grazing but is completely aware of its surroundings. In other words, you cannot sneak up on a deer because its awareness is very high and if your intentions are to hurt it, it will run away. Spiritually speaking, when you are clear of the distractions of the world, you will gain understanding of how this world works. Thus, nothing can surprise you because you will feel that something is about to happen before it occurs. When you have a high awareness you will understand your daily interactions better."

Yutian: "Awareness is the knowledge of the existence of something. It doesn't have to be physical. It can be emotional, spiritual or virtual."

According to Bob Proctor, 7 levels of Awareness exist, beginning with # 7. As you gain greater insight, you reach #1, the highest level or Mastery. They are:

1. **"Mastery-** respond, think and plan.
2. **Experience-** your new actions change your RESULTS.
3. **Discipline-** you give yourself a command and follow it.
4. **Individual-** you express your uniqueness.
5. **Aspiration-** you desire something greater.
6. **Mass-** follow the masses (follow your paradigms).
7. **Animal-** re-act: fight or flight."

Before a baby begins walking, the baby is aware of his/her surroundings and acts with faith. The baby doesn't attempt to walk and stop when it falls. Instead, the baby falls; stands up; takes a number of steps and falls again, repeating the process until mastery (walking) is achieved.

Humanity, in their adult bodies, is conditioned to stop when the 'perception' of failure occurs. It is with greater awareness of the mind; thoughts and conditioning, that humanity may regain its power. To expand in awareness means to grow, in all ways, both comfortable and uncomfortable.

As Gay Hendricks stated, "If you expand to the fullness of yourself, it gives other people permission to expand to their fullness."

Are you aware of how what goes into your mind while you watch TV affects you? Are you aware that everything is energy and the words emanating from the TV carry energy that goes into your cells? Thich Nhat Hanh states "We turn on the TV and leave it on, allowing someone else to guide us, shape us and destroy us. We must be aware of which programs do harm to our nervous system, minds and hearts and which programs benefit us."

Daily, you are abundantly choosing. What choices will you allow? What do you do with your free time? Will you embrace yourself, in your perfection, beauty and power as you are or will you limit your world by living in a lower frequency of your perception of negativity and impossibility? As Dr. Deepak Chopra stated "Desires are fulfilled according to your level of awareness. When awareness is pure, every desire is fulfilled completely."

"The struggle is inner: Chicano, Indio, American Indian, mojado, mexicano, immigrant Latino, Anglo in power, working class Anglo, Black, Asian--our psyches resemble the border towns and are populated by the same people. The struggle has always been inner and is played out in outer terrains. Awareness of our situation must come before inner changes, which in turn come before changes in society. Nothing happens in the "real" world unless it first happens in the images in our heads." Gloria Anzaldua, Tejana Chicana poet

Invitation to expand:
I invite you to review the above questions *before and after* reading this book. What level of awareness do you vibrate from? What feelings, thoughts come up for you? How did your awareness increase? What do you attribute it to? How do you feel?

Meditate on the following story Osho shared, entitled *The Goose Is Out*. A small goose was placed in a bottle and fed, growing larger and larger so it could not get out of the bottle. A Master told the disciple to bring the goose out without killing the goose or destroying the bottle. How did the disciple do this?

After ruminating about it, the disciple understands the story is a reflection of the mind and awareness. The bottle is the mind and the goose is you. The disciple told the Master the goose is out. The Master replied "You understood it. Now keep it out. It has never been in." In other words, the goose is awareness and mind represents the thoughts you observe on your brain's screen (bottle). Awareness (the goose) is not in the bottle (the mind). Awareness has always been outside of the mind. Osho suggests creating a distance between you and your mind, viewing it as you would a film.

BELIEFS

"To master your thoughts and imagination and therefore your life and destiny, you must first master their captain- your beliefs."
Mike Dooley

Earlier, we mentioned Bob Proctor's definition of attitude being the sum of your thoughts, feelings and actions. Beliefs determine what thoughts occur and then feelings and actions follow. Mike Dooley also expressed "Whenever you catch yourself expressing an opinion, in thought; word or deed, realize you've just nailed a belief that's busy building your life around you." What beliefs did you build your life around? How do they serve you? Are they serving you?

Peggy McColl states "You don't need to know the "how"; you just need to have faith and keep moving towards your goal. The rest will be revealed to you." When you drive down the road, although you see in front of you, you cannot see 1 mile ahead of you. Reaching your goals is similar. You cannot see the goal occurring until it happens, thus, belief and action propel it forward. Iyanla Vanzant stated "Be willing to believe there is another way." Be willing to embrace the uncertainty with faith and knowing that your beliefs will come to fruition.

Mike Dooley stated, "Your beliefs permit or deny your dreams." Remember Dooley's statement when your negative thoughts begin, or as a friend, Louie says "the itty bitty shitty committee" takes over. Turn off this committee forever. If you do not know how, you will when you finish this book.

BODY (PHYSICAL)

The human body has "**24,000 fibers in the ear; 500 muscles; 200 bones and 7 miles of nerve fibers. The brain contains 13 billion nerve cells. Within the cells are 1 thousand billion proteins; 4 million pain sensitive structures and 500 touch detectors.**" Og Mandino, *The Greatest Miracle in the World*

Bob Proctor shares that "Most people take better care of their car than their body." Unlike regular car maintenance, many people fail to apply regular care to their bodies, neglecting to nourish them with nutrients, movement and preventative care. However, your bodies, the magnificent machines they are, continue running.

In *The Integral Vision*, Ken Wilber mentions that you have three bodies, a gross body, subtle body and causal body. The gross body refers to the physical, material and sensorimotor body. This is the body in a waking state of awareness. The subtle body includes light, energy, emotional feelings and flowing images. This is the dream state when the mind and soul touch other souls and are not bound by sensory reality. The third body, the casual body (a formless body), is a deep sleep state (can be entered into fully aware) and an infinite energetic body from which all possibilities exist.

Invitation to expand:

What if, daily, you treated your body as the beautiful and powerful gem it is? What if you spoke lovingly to it and cared for it like you care for a newborn child- with love, positive attention and appreciation? What if you stopped abusing it with toxins and chemically produced junk?

WHAT IF YOU ASKED YOUR BODY WHAT IT NEEDED TO NOURISH YOUR HEART, MIND AND SOUL AND TOOK CONSISTENT ACTION? What if it is THAT easy? Perhaps your body responds by embracing you in a loving cocoon of health; favorite memories; nutrient rich food and the most beautiful and bountiful abundance. Is this experiment worth it? It was for me. Try it and share your story with me.

BREATH/BREATHING

"3 deep breaths transform body chemistry of fear into the body chemistry of excitement."
Gay Hendricks, Ph.D.

In *The Art of Breathing*, Nancy Zi shares 30 exercises of chi yi, based on chi kung or the ancient Chinese art of breath manipulation. She states that "Controlled deep breathing helps the body transform the air we breathe into energy. The mind, coordinated with breathing, can be responsible for the state of one's physical health, one's blood pressure, one's immune system and one's mental condition."

One type of exercise, an imagery drill, includes an exercise called Eyedropper. Stand tall and relaxed. Imagine you are an upside down eyedropper. Squeeze bulb and air is squeezed out. Release bulb and air is taken into body. Now imagine opening glass tube ends where the back of the nose and throat meet. Let air flow in and out through this opening. Apply this image as you breathe naturally to help you with abdominal breathing.

Another exercise relieves throbbing pain. 1) Take deep, full inhalations and lingering, thorough exhalations. 2) Focus your mind on throbbing pains. Monitor them by mentally counting as you continue with chi yi (exhalation/inhalation) breathing. Count 1-4 or 1-10. Repeat sequence. 3) Continue to count. You will notice pain subsiding and throbs becoming regular and painless.

Nancy Zi offers the following 6 lessons to guide you through the imagery drills and breathing exercises: 1) Leading the breath (think of exhalation/inhalation) instead of reverse. This will produce no audible sound. 2) Coordinating the breath enables muscles to grow sensitive and responsive. 3) Controlling the breath allows the abdominal deep breathing application to improve breathing. 4) Varying and extending the breath. 5) Using breath to develop the Core. 6) Applying the breath to develop deeper Core awareness (decrease negative emotions, pain, fear, depression, etc.). Apply to all activities patiently and persistently.

CALMNESS OF MIND

Napoleon Hill wrote a powerful classic, *As A Man Thinketh*. In it, he devotes a chapter to calmness of mind. He begins the chapter with: "Calmness of mind is one of the beautiful jewels of wisdom. It is the result of long and patient effort in self-control. Its presence is an indication of ripened experience and of a more than ordinary knowledge of the laws and operations of thought. The more tranquil a man becomes, the greater is his success, his influence, his power for good."

The laws Napoleon Hill refers to are the Universal Laws (see UNIVERSAL LAWS). I highly encourage you to own *As A Man Thinketh,* continually studying it, one paragraph or chapter at a time.

CELLS

"Upon the union of the male germ cell with the female egg cell, a new cell is created which almost immediately splits into two parts. One of these grows rapidly, creating the human body of the individual with all its organs and dies only with the individual."
Christian Lous Lange

Ann Wigmore, author of *The Wheatgrass Book*, mentioned "Each of us is a keeper of over ten trillion little batteries called cells. Like flashlight batteries, our cells hold a charge of electricity. In order for this charge to be strong and steady, we need to have a steady supply of proper nutrients." She lists wheatgrass as a key ingredient. (See Wheatgrass section). For you to enjoy health and vitality, your cells must be nourished and fed with positive, life affirming food, thoughts and actions. Cells are often called the building blocks of life.

In addition to physical nutrients from food, life affirming thoughts are vital. Dr. Bruce Lipton, expert cell biologist and author states that your paradigm of cell control may need an overhaul. In his book, *Spontaneous Evolution,* he states that the previously held belief in genetic control or genes controlling life is incorrect. In this model you were victims because you couldn't change genes. The new science states genes are controlled via epigenetic control, or control above genes. In other words, genes are controlled by your response to environment. Therefore, if you change your environment, the cell activity changes. Whether your environment is toxic or healthy, the genes respond accordingly and promote disease or health. However, you are in control and powerful as you choose your environment. He suggests you focus on the NOW and create habits that shift your thoughts. Guiliana Conforto, author of *Man's Cosmic Game* reiterates Dr. Lipton's research sharing "Every cell pulsates, absorbs, reflects and interacts with the acoustic oscillations of the medium."

Invitation to expand:
Everything in this book speaks of empowering yourself with knowledge and altering your inner and outer environment. When your paradigms, or set of beliefs change, your cells change. As you read, I invite you to detach from your former knowledge, embracing the words you read with a new understanding of what it means to think- linking science with spirituality. May you affectionately hug the science and esoteric connection and truly grasp that you are the Master of your fate!

CHAKRAS

In her book, *Wheels of Life*, Anodea Judith, Ph.D., defines chakra as "An organizational center for the reception, assimilation and transmission of life energy." Each of the 7 chakras corresponds to 7 basic levels of consciousness; various types of activity; stages in personal and cultural life cycles and patterns of consciousness (belief systems).

She states that each chakra is associated with a body part and color. Chakra 1 is located at the base of the spine and associated with survival and the color red, like strawberries. Chakra 2 is in the lower abdomen and associated with emotions and sexuality and the color orange, like oranges. Personal power, self-esteem, will and the color yellow (like the sun) are associated with the third Chakra, in the solar plexus. The fourth Chakra is near the sternum and is associated with love and green, the color of grass. Chakra 5 is in the throat and associated with creativity and communication and the color blue, like turquoise or a tropical sea. The middle of the forehead (3rd eye) houses Chakra 6 and this center involves intuition, imagination and clairvoyance and the color lavender. Chakra 7 is on the top of the head and is associated with understanding, wisdom, heaven and the color of a diamond.

GRATEFUL FOR THE CHALLENGES

"Be grateful for the challenges as they enrich your soul's lessons."
Pagona

Stephen R. Covey shared that "Opposition is a natural part of life. Just as we develop our physical muscles through overcoming opposition-such as lifting weights-we develop our character muscles by overcoming challenges and adversity." By embracing your challenges, you remain open to your life's lessons and stay in a higher vibration.

Invitation to expand:
Reflect on your life and notice challenges you overcame. What were they and what did you learn from them? How did they shape who you are?

EMBRACING CHANGE

"True change is always made at the level of "being" not "doing."
Neale Donald Walsch in *Conversations With God, Book III*

In her book, *Your Destiny Switch*, Peggy McColl shared "The ability to change your life comes from the power of love in your heart. Love connects you to your other positive emotions. It's the ultimate source of emotional fuel, so plug into it." Change is inevitable and you must flow, like a river flowing upstream or downstream with whatever comes your way, no matter what it does or does not look like. Love makes change easier, especially love for oneself and humanity. Embrace the annual, daily and hourly changes trusting that the Universe is working with you, unfolding greatness and opportunities. Gail Sheehy stated "If we don't change we don't grow. If we don't grow we aren't really living."

CHARACTER

"A man is literally what he thinks, his character being the complete sum of all his thoughts."
James Allen

According to Alphonse Karr, "Every man has 3 characters: that which he exhibits, that which he has and that which he thinks he has." Think about the person you exhibit to the world- what is he/she like? How about the person you think you are? What is that person like? Now imagine the person you are-what does that person do, how does that person spend his/her time? What type of books does that person read? Does that person read or prefer to watch TV? Embrace the real character of who you are, the beautiful and not so gorgeous aspects of you.

Invitation to expand:
The word character is a French word- *caractere* which means imprint on the soul. "Character is revealed when our mask is removed." Remove the masks you hide behind and you will reveal yourself to you. These masks may be unknown facades and may require inner work. This work will improve your life, if you are willing and open to it. Remember Lakota Tiokasin Ghosthorse words "Real eyes realize real lies." Keep this in mind when the lies you tell yourself about who you are pop up. Be true to you and embrace everything about you.

CHI- "THE THREAD CONNECTING ALL THINGS"

Chi/qi is used interchangeably and means "air" or "breath" in Chinese. Through meditation, Taoists discovered Chi as a subtle electromagnetic force flowing in the body. In Chinese Medicine, chi follows unseen pathways called meridians.

According to Ted Kaptchuk, in *The Web That Has No Weaver,* "qi is the thread connecting all things; qi is the potential and actualization of transformation; qi is the fundamental quality of being and becoming." Kaptchuk also states that "Qi does not "cause" change. Qi is present before, during and after the transformation."

In the text, *Foundations of Chinese Medicine*, the author, Giovanni Maciocia stated "Just as Qi is the material substratum of the universe, it is also the material and spiritual substratum of human life." He continues in the "Classic of Difficulties," with Qi's definition as "The root of a human being. Qi is an energy that manifests simultaneously on the physical and spiritual level. Qi is in a constant state of flux and in varying states of aggregation. When it condenses, energy transforms and accumulates into physical shape." Although Qi is one universal energy, it assumes different forms and functions. In Chinese Medicine, Qi has two major aspects. It nourishes the mind and body and indicates the functional activity of the internal organs.

CHOICE/DECISIONS

"Every second we choose to nourish ourselves in a way that supports or depletes our lives and to think and speak about other people in a way that is honoring or dishonoring. What choice are you going to make today?"
Gregg Braden, author of *The Divine Matrix*

What dictates choice? In *Conversations With God, Book I,* Neale Donald Walsch mentions that what dictates all choice is "Who and What you think you are and Who and What you choose to be." How do you answer these 2 questions?

Mary Morrissey tells you "Make 1 decision daily to talk, read and think about your dream." How would this one decision impact your dream? How would this change your life? According to Bob Proctor, "You are the only problem you will ever have and you are the only solution. Change is inevitable, personal growth is always a personal decision."

If you operate from a place of worry and stress and believe you have no choice, your perception of what you can accomplish will be limited. Stress causes the body to shut down and become unreceptive to the good, the wisdom and opportunities around you. Maureen Killoran states "Stress is not what happens to us. It's our response TO what happens. And RESPONSE is something we can choose." We choose our responses daily. How are you choosing? Are you living in an indecisive world or are you making conscious quick choices daily? Napoleon Hill states "Indecision is the seedling of fear." Let's motivate you to make quick decisions based on intuition that can be changed, if needed, along the way.

Og Mandino, in his book, *The Greatest Miracle in The World* invites you to:

"Choose to laugh ... rather than cry

Choose to persevere ... rather than quit

Choose to praise ... rather than gossip

Choose to love ... rather than hate

Choose to act ... rather than procrastinate

Choose to pray ... rather than curse

Choose to live ... rather than die

Choose to grow ... rather than rot

Choose to create ... rather than destroy

Choose to heal ... rather than wound."

Invitation to expand:

The power of choice is yours daily. When you have a choice to make, center yourself in a calm space as it often difficult to make decisions while worried, stressed or anxious. Ask what is the best and highest good for you? Trust the first answer you receive, even if you do not know how or why it came. This is your intuition directing your choice.

Another option is my preferred way to make decisions. In his program Success Puzzle, Bob Proctor suggests asking the following 4 questions when faced with a decision: 1) Do I want to be/do/have this? 2) Will being/doing/having this move me in the direction of my goal? 3) Is being/doing or having this in harmony with God's laws or Universal Laws? 4) Will being/doing this violate the rights of others? Ask yourself these 4 questions and you will make decisions quickly. Proctor also taught that successful people make decisions quickly and are slow to change them.

COMMITMENT

"Until one is committed, there is hesitancy, the chance to draw

back, always ineffectiveness. **Concerning all acts of initiative and creation, there is one elementary truth, the ignorance of which kills countless ideas and splendid plans: that the moment one definitely commits oneself, then providence moves too. A whole stream of events issues from the decision, raising in one's favor all manner of unforeseen incidents, meetings and material assistance, which no man could have dreamt would have come his way."**

W.H. Murray, during one of his Himalayan expeditions

In *Secrets of the Millionaire Mind*, T. Harv Eker mentions commitment. He states that to commit is to "devote oneself unreservedly." Unreservedly means you put 100% into it. He also makes a great distinction about 'I want', 'I choose' and 'I commit.' Wanting, he states may not lead to having and wanting without having leads to wanting. Choosing has a stronger energy while committing has the highest energy.

Invitation to expand:
Look at what are you committed to. How does it serve you? What are you willing to change and give 100% of yourself towards achieving? Think of what you commit to now. Write down what you will commit to. For example, I commit to being compassionate; healthy; happy; prosperous; successful; loving and open.

COMPASSION

Dr. Deepak Chopra, in his book, *The Path to Love*, offers the following code for compassion:
"Be kind to yourself and others.
Come from love every moment you can.
Speak of love with others. Remind each other of your spiritual purpose.
Never give up hope.
Know that you are loved."

Ram Dass and Mirabai Bush, in their book *Compassion in Action: Setting Out on The Path of Service,* share that the meaning of compassion was first mentioned in: The Bible, Koran, Dhammapada, Bhagavad Gita, Ramayana, Tao Te Ching and Popul Vuh. They state "Compassion in action is paradoxical and is done for others but nurtures the self." When you are compassionate, you open your heart to suffering and sadness, anger and all emotions. Compassion begins with every being and brings with it awakening, helping humanity.

Dass and Bush state "Compassion is the basis for all truthful relationships: it means being present with love- for ourselves and for all life, including animals, fish, birds and trees. Compassion is bringing our deepest truth into our actions."

Invitation to expand:

I invite you to reflect upon 2 questions Ram Dass asked: What are the roots of your caring action? What do you have to offer to alleviate another's suffering?

COMPLAINING/COMPLAINTS

"When you are complaining, you become a living, breathing crap magnet."
Anonymous

According to Eckhart Tolle, complaining is a form of non-acceptance. Like the above quote, complaining puts you in a negative vibration. In his book, *The Secrets of The Millionaire Mind,* T. Harv Eker suggests that for 1 week, you choose not to complain (out loud or in your head). Notice how your week progressed and what changes occurred. How do you feel and what did you attract into your life? The action you wish to take will be from insight and not negativity, including complaining.

SOUL INGREDIENTS

CONSCIOUSNESS

"Without a connection to Consciousness, people are condemned to 'the box'-the vibrational 'box' of limited and bewildered perception."
David Icke

Neale Donald Walsch in *Conversations With God, Book III* states "You have to raise consciousness before you can change consciousness." He says it is wise to choose the company of high consciousness beings. He also mentions you always have the following 3 choices in life: 1) Allowing uncontrolled thoughts to create The Moment 2) Allowing creative consciousness to create The Moment and 3) Allowing collective consciousness to create The Moment. Which will you choose?

Daily you have many opportunities to raise your consciousness. One way to raise your consciousness is to increase your intelligence. Another way is to examine what your current reality is. In other words, what do you perceive as your reality? When you change your perception, your reality changes. A third way is to resolve disagreements. According to Dr. Deepak Chopra "All disagreements are results of misunderstanding someone else's level of consciousness." You can also embrace each another and raise your frequency of love. Most importantly, you must change how you are being to change how you are doing. Living with infinite compassion and gratitude will change your consciousness.

Invitation to expand:
What are you conscious of? What is not in your consciousness? Why? What is keeping you from that knowing?

COURAGE

"Courage is not the absence of fear, rather the judgment that something else is more important than fear."
Ambrose Redmoon

36

Judith Orloff, MD reminds you that "To awaken is an act of courage." When you work on yourself, you awaken to the Divine within and allow things like the illusions of fear, lack; limitation, etc. to gently leave your body, energy field and surroundings.

Like Redmoon, Nelson Mandela spoke about the relationship of courage and fear. He stated "I learned that courage was not the absence of fear, but the triumph over it. The brave man is not he who does not feel afraid, but he who conquers that fear." Remember that fear is an illusion (created in your mind) and it can be conquered. Your state of mind is tremendously powerful. Ask anyone, who like me, practices Bikram yoga for 90 minutes, in a room heated to 105 °F with 40% humidity. They will attest to the power of courage and the mind.

Barbara De Angelis reminds you that "True transformation requires great acts of courage. It is not courage to do things. Great courage is not about getting or doing, it's about relinquishing, letting go and shifting your identification." Daily courage entails pushing through your 'perceived' obstacles, embracing your inner power.

Invitation to expand:
In the film, The *Edge of Never,* one of the main characters asked a vital question: "Do you have the courage to take complete responsibility for every choice and fully embrace every moment?" How do you answer that question?

CREATE/CREATIVITY/CREATOR

"You are the absolute creator of what happens to you. This means now...there is awesome power in knowing this fact. As long as there is one tiny part of you that thinks the world is doing it to you, the world is going to do it to you. When you know 100% that you create it, you start influencing the world around you in a much bigger and more positive way."
Gay Hendricks, Ph.D.

You are all gifted with creativity at birth, whether you acknowledge this or not. Peter Koestenbaum stated "Creativity is harnessing universality and making it flow through your eyes." Creativity is like intuition; some developed and practice it daily while others allow it to remain dormant. Everyone is creative yet some forgot it while others embrace and express it. Remember when you were a child- creativity flowed through you with ease. Napoleon Hill stated that "Creativity is being able to see what everybody else has seen and think what nobody else has thought so that you can do what nobody else has done."

Julian Cameron, in her book, *Artist's Way*, lists the basic principles of creativity. They include: 1) "Creativity is the natural order of life. Life is pure creative energy. 2) We are creations and are meant to continue creativity by being creative ourselves. 3) Our creative dreams and yearnings come from a divine source. As we move toward our dreams, we move toward our divinity."

DANCE

"If you can walk you can dance. If you can talk you can sing."
Zimbabwe Proverb

Martha Graham stated "Dance is the hidden language of the soul of the body." Dancing encourages moving to your rhythm and awakening. For me, dancing is like energy healing; lovemaking and vibrant, healthy, perfectly seasoned food rolled into one. It is pure joy and freedom simultaneously. I like to say "Dancing makes my cells explode with laughter."

Rabbi Miriyam Glazer said "I believe you can get to know someone really well on the dance floor, just by dancing with them." Dancing is an invitation and a way of expressing without spoken word.

Dance is also ancient practice. One of the most important rites of passage is the sacred Lakota Tribe Sun Dance to Wakan Tanka, the Great Spirit. For the Sufi followers of Rumi, the Whirling Dervishes, 800 year old ritualized dances, bring the dancer closer to an ecstatic union with the Divine.

More people are realizing dancing solo is the beginning of awakening self-knowledge, self-awareness and soul-healing, leading to spiritual awakening. Gabrielle Roth expressed the realization of the "One" and the "Many" with the following: "Sweat is holy water, prayer beads, pearls of liquid that release your past. Sweat is an ancient and universal form of self-healing, whether done in the gym, the sauna or the sweat lodge. The more you dance, the more you sweat. The more you sweat, the more you pray. The more you pray, the closer you come to ecstasy."

Other examples of dance include Anna Halprin's, Dance of Liberation™ (DOL). DOL integrates shamanic journeying, breath work, drumming, global music, sweat lodges and fasting to eliminate physical, mental, emotional and spiritual blocks.

Invitation to expand:

I invite you to dance, to release the 'I have no rhythm' or 'I can't dance' paradigms and embrace your soul's soul. It may not be the most perfect hip hop, salsa, techno or waltz, yet it will be that which transforms you. This is in gratitude to my dear friend Christine Harmon Tangishaka, for your wisdom, compassion and of course, dance skills, propelled me in my dance of liberation.

What is your dance? Focus on your body flowing to the rhythm and how happy your body feels with each movement. Bring attention to your heart, allowing yourself total freedom from thought. What is your soul's favorite tune? Hear it, feel it and most importantly, as songwriters Mark D. Sanders and Tia Sillers wrote in the I Hope You Dance lyrics, "When you get the chance to sit it out or dance, I hope you dance."

DIALOGUE

"The most important aspect of freedom of speech is freedom to learn. All education is a continuous dialogue-questions and answers that pursue every problem on the horizon. That is the essence of academic freedom."
William Orville Douglas

Dialogue and honest, compassionate communication is extremely important, especially in this technological society. Without open communication and acceptance of different opinions and ways of being, society and humanity have difficulty thriving. Without dialogue, resolution cannot occur.

Marie Curie expressed "Nothing is to be feared. It is only to be understood." Like Curie's words, nothing, including dialogue and open, honest communication needs to be feared. Instead, it must be embraced. When dialogue is embraced, deep introspection and healing can begin. It begins on an individual level first and then on a global level.

DISCERNMENT

"Exchanging our mortal intelligence for divine intelligence, we begin to see beyond appearances."
Marianne Williamson, from *The Gift of Change: Spiritual Guidance for Living Your Best Life*

Mary Morrissey states "Pay attention to what you are paying attention to." When doing this, your habits can be changed quicker than without your awareness of what you give attention to. Discernment allows you to stay in touch with your higher self and live and operate from a place of higher integrity, authenticity and love. With discernment one gains clarity and a higher purpose for living. I like to think of it as seeing the true, divine nature of everyone. When you recognize everyone operates the best they can with what they have, a space for understanding and forgiveness opens.

Sue Singleton, co-founder and medical intuitive at The Way to Balance, www.thewaytobalance.com, stated discernment is "The ability to determine or recognize accurately, to truly know truth. It is the opposite of judgment and includes justice, kindness, honesty and power to say "No."

The Singletons taught me about discernment years ago in the Energy of Life Process (EOL). I learned to ask two questions to help discern anything anywhere. Note that this is a simplified view of the process and depending on where you are on your journey; you may require more or less practice and more or less understanding of the protocols.

First, ask What is for my highest good to know about this _____ (insert topic)? Second, ask Would it be for my highest good to use/buy, etc. _____ (insert topic)? Trust the first answer that comes to you. If you do not receive an immediate answer, continue asking clarifying questions. For example, while reading a scientific article about krill oil, I asked, What is for my highest good to know about this oil? My response was it is a rich Omega 3 source. The next question asked was, Is it for my highest good to use this oil? The response was no. When I inquired further, I was told it contains mercury. This is one example of how these two questions can be used to discern anything. Remember to discern means to think and act spontaneously, trusting information that instantly comes to you.

DIVINE CONSCIOUSNESS

"[Christ consciousness might be seen as] The divine consciousness that was in Jesus and is in you and me, a radically, all-inclusive consciousness of Light, Love and Life that is resurrected from the stream of time upon the death of the loveless and self-contracting ego, revealing a destiny beyond death, beyond suffering, beyond space and time and tears and terror."
Ken Wilber, *The Integral Vision*

What is divine consciousness? In his book, *The Integral Vision,* Ken Wilber stated over the last 300 years, researchers learned that "You interpret any spiritual (meditative, altered) state of consciousness according to your stage of consciousness." In other words, you see what you see according to the level of your conscious development.

How can divine consciousness be attained? When you operate from the heart, continuously shining your light, love and compassion in the world, you live in divine consciousness. Dr. Zhi Gang Sha, in his book *The Power of Soul,* shares that divine consciousness can be attained by following 7 steps: Offer soul healing; prevent sickness of the soul; soul rejuvenation; soul transformation; enlighten humanity and then enlighten all souls.

According to the Bhagavad Gita "He whose happiness is within, whose contentment is within, whose light is all within, that yogi, being one with Brahman, attains eternal freedom in divine consciousness." If inner peace reigns in one's heart and the above 7 steps are attained, one may reach a higher consciousness, one of divine consciousness.

SOUL INGREDIENTS

Kryon stated it is about the knowledge of the God inside you (the ancients). You are here to understand and embrace this knowledge inside you. This creates light on the planet. Know you are loved, perfect and whole EXACTLY as you are, as you sit, stand, drive or run; in the space you call home, work or solitude. You are perfect, a reflection of the Divine.

How I longed to hear and truly grasp these words at an earlier age. That longing continues to feed my thirst for knowledge and wisdom. How I wish for you, dear reader to embrace the Divinity you call you. Do not allow one moment to pass without embracing the true you, realizing your soul has many ingredients, some you may never have heard of. Which will you disregard and which will you embrace?

DNA

"DNA is the antenna of the body, listening for the profundities of your epiphanies, the breakthroughs in the tight fabric of fear and frustration. It measures the heights of your joy, the peaks of your passion, and sees the smile as you finally understand that the pathway to God has always been open and available to you. It responds by orchestrating cellular structure to enhance who you are and to complement your life on Earth."
Kryon in *The Twelve Layers of DNA*

Growing up in America's public school system, I learned that DNA is made up of 2 spiral strands composed of A-T-C-G base pairs. Much thought was not given to the metaphysical properties of DNA. At that time, The Human Genome project was not conceived and little was known of "junk" DNA.

In *Twelve Layers of DNA*, DNA researcher Dr. Todd Ovokaitys mentioned an experiment by Russian physicist Vladimir Poponin that measured light polarization and light orientation states (photons). Poponin noted that light waves moved randomly. When he placed DNA within a study chamber and measured the photons, he found light waves organized in a coherent pattern. This was a surprise to him and he indicated, "DNA produced a powerful field that strongly organized the space around it."

When Poponin removed the DNA, he noticed that the photons remained in the same organized pattern. Again, this suggested "There remained a potent residual effect in the space because DNA occupied that space." Dr. Todd shared that this "phantom DNA effect" and the 97% of Human Genome considered noncoding "junk" leave many unsolved DNA mysteries. Below I address some of these mysteries according to Kryon.

In *Twelve Layers of DNA*, Kryon suggested DNA is multidimensional with 12 energy 'layers'. Simply stated, Layer 1 is the physical double helix. Layer 2 represents a search for the human's life lessons. Layer 3 is called the Ascension and Activation layer because it listens for consciousness changes. Layers 4 and 5 are the "the essence of your expression (this specific life on Earth) and your divinity on the planet." Layer 6, or the "I AM" layer, represents communication with God through prayer and meditation. Layer 7 is "a divine revelation layer, the metaphor of which is the end of innocence and the beginning of spiritual awareness." Layer 8 is interdimensional or in a quantum state and the "personal Akashic Record of the core soul." Layer 9, the healing layer is also multidimensional. Chinese Medicine and kinesiology work with this layer of the body's awareness. It is dormant until spoken to. Layers 10-12 are divine God layers. Layer 10 begins "a Human's search for God." Layer 11 is the divine feminine energy that needs to be called upon and "activated with compassionate events on the planet." Layer 12 is involved in all 11 layers and the "creator energy within your DNA.

DREAM/DREAMS

"There is only one thing that makes a dream impossible to achieve: the fear of failure."
Paulo Coelho, author of *The Alchemist*

Courage and fear were discussed above and now dreams and courage are addressed. To live a dream, you must exhibit courage. As Sigmund Freud once stated, "Dreams are often most profound when they seem the most crazy." Many people may regard you as crazy when you mention your dreams. Bob Proctor advised us to keep dreams to ourselves and share with only those who support us in achieving them. You must realize every worthwhile endeavor begins with a dream. Be it large or small, a dream propels you to accomplish bigger and better things. John Assaraf and Murray Smith told you "Every billionaire begins as a child with a dream."

Invitation to expand:
What are your dreams? How will you achieve them? Notice the people in your life who, when you share your dreams roll their eyes or offer statements like that's crazy. Perhaps you limit your interactions with them. Become like George Bernard Shaw when he said "Some men see things as they are and ask "Why?" I dream of things that never were and say, "Why not?" Remember the words of Tony Gaskins, "If you don't build your dream, someone will hire you to help build theirs."

EDUCATION

"Leaders are as much students as those who follow them. Life for us is an eternal school. There is a Dagara saying: "Each person is a student. If you stop learning you must stop existing." Questions followers bring to leaders lead them to new places, where they find answers they didn't have before."
Sobonfu E. Somé, in *Falling Out of Grace*

Biologist, Thomas H. Huxley stated it well with the words "Perhaps the most valuable result of all education is the ability to make yourself do the thing you have to do, when it ought to be done, whether you like it or not. It is the first lesson that ought to be learned and however early a man's training begins, it is probably the last lesson that he learns thoroughly." How many learned this lesson? If you did not, why? This is a very important part of discipline and getting things done. To train to become an acupuncturist; astronaut; athlete; musician; salesperson; teacher or whatever you desire, daily education and action must occur. This is a common trait shared by all successful people I know and is repeatedly emphasized.

In *Book II of Conversations With God,* Neale Donald Walsch suggests that schools may wish to teach value based education encouraging questions and concepts instead of subjects. Classes could be taught in the following concepts: Understanding Power; Ethical Economics; Celebrating Self, Valuing Others and Honesty and Responsibility and Listening.

Mike Adams, Health Ranger once wrote "Education transforms an ordinary, closed minded human being into a world citizen." These words stuck with me through exams and difficult days in my formal education. Think of what your education taught you. Now think of what it didn't teach you, find that and teach yourself. In the words of Arthur W. Hummel, former Head, Division of Orientalia Library of Congress, Washington, D.C. 1962, "The world has a place for humility, yielding, gentleness and serenity. To enjoy these benefits, one must learn to unlearn one's learning."

EMBRACE

"In many cultures, including the Dagara, the idea is you sculpt your face as you live and each wrinkle shows a particular joy or pain you survived. You would never have a facelift to look younger or color your hair when it turns gray. That would be a loss of beauty, a loss of grace."
Sobonfu E. Somé

Invitation to expand:
What do you need to embrace? What needs hugging that you are not embracing? It is your body, your relationships, your career, your home? Why are you resisting it? Take 1 action step daily toward embracing it and you may find that you needed embracing. Watch the film *What the Bleep Do We Know?* for a beautiful example of embracing self. Read Dalai Lama's books for profound demonstrations of embracing, empathy and equanimity. Learn to love all parts of yourself, including the 'unlovable' ones and embrace the beauty and perfection that is you.

EMOTIONAL WELLNESS

In *Emotional Wellness*, Osho shares "Emotions cannot be permanent. That's why they are called "emotions"-the word comes from "motion," movement. They move, hence, they are "emotions." From one to another you continually change."

How do you attain emotional wellness? Osho states that acceptance, watchfulness, understanding your emotional types and not suppressing anything are crucial. Acceptance involves moving with nature, feeling that you are coming and going, like a wave. Watchfulness entails becoming aware while the act occurs, remembering before the act (when it is in your mind) and lastly, "To catch hold of this process, which results in an act, before it becomes a thought. Feeling comes first, then thought, then comes the act." Understanding your emotional types involves knowing whether you are head oriented, heart oriented or body oriented. Head oriented people have difficulty having feelings and praying. Heart oriented people feel more than they think while body oriented people love active methods and not silent ones. Lastly, expression, instead of repression is critical. A suppression example is suppressed anger that over a period of time becomes depression.

Osho also offers exercises to embrace emotional wellness including: transforming fear; feeling your pain and moving to the opposite of your feeling. To transform fear, Osho suggests not calling it fear. He suggests eliminating names for things like fear, sadness, etc. and instead watching the emotions arising. To feel your pain involves being thankful, for ex. that someone hurt you as that person gave you an opportunity to feel a wound. Moving to the opposite of your feelings entails doing something to break the habit. For example, instead of being sad, create a new habit of being happy. It gets easier with practice.

Invitation to expand:
Are you head oriented, heart oriented, body oriented or a combination? How can this knowledge empower you? What does embracing emotional wellness look like for you?

EMPATHY

"My knowledge of myself is direct, synthetic, from within outwards; my knowledge of other persons is indirect, analytical, from outside inwards. My knowledge of myself starts at the core; that of others at the crust."
Salvador de Madariaga, *Essays with a Purpose*

C. JoyBell stated "Our bodies have five senses: touch, smell, taste, sight and hearing. Not to be overlooked are the senses of our souls: intuition, peace, foresight, trust and empathy. The differences between people lie in their use of these senses; most people don't know anything about the inner senses while a few people rely on them as they rely on their physical senses and probably more." What if you more often engaged the senses of your soul (intuition, peace, foresight, trust and empathy) as C. JoyBell stated? What would your life be like?

Empathy is a precursor to happiness, love and peace. Without it, you live in a self- absorbed bubble, unable to relate to worldly occurrences, cultures, unfamiliar food, customs or philosophies. How can learning occur if empathy is non- existent? Part of learning involves understanding others without being in their situation. It involves embracing yourself and every other self, especially the 'ugly' selves. Empathy is happily married to equanimity, discussed below. As Roger Ebert stated, "I believe empathy is the most essential quality of civilization."

ENCOURAGEMENT

"If I could give you one thought, it would be to lift someone up. Lift a stranger up--lift her up. I would ask you, mother and father, brother and sister, lovers, mother and daughter, father and son, lift someone. The very idea of lifting someone up will lift you, as well."
Maya Angelou

Surround yourself with people who encourage you. Encourage them and allow yourself to grow. Encourage yourself and believe that you are capable of everything and anything.

ENERGY

How many times did you hear Lavoisier, a French chemist's words "Nothing is created, nothing is destroyed?" If you have not, it may be a good idea to take note. A fundamental truth may be used to understand yourself better as you too, are made of energy. Since everything is made of energy and energy is neither created nor destroyed, this gives a new perspective on many illusions, including life and death.

Neale Donald Walsch, in *Conversations With God, Book I* shared that "Emotion is energy in motion, When you move energy, you create effect. If you move enough energy, you create matter. Matter is energy conglomerated. Every Master understands this law. It is the alchemy of the universe. It is the secret of all life."

Invitation to expand:
Neale Donald Walsch also stated, *In Conversations With God, Book I* "Thought is pure energy. The energy of your thought never dies. It leaves your being and heads out into the universe, extending forever." I discuss thoughts in their own section and invite you to tune into the energy of your thoughts, family, surroundings and work environment. Take the opportunity to observe your feelings when you walk into a room and when you leave. Notice the energy when you meet a friend, make love, cook, laugh, dance and relax. Use every chance to witness energy- both with your eyes open and closed. You will be amazed at your findings.

EQUANIMITY

"Equanimity is characterized as promoting neutrality toward all beings. Its function is to see equality in beings. It is manifested as the quieting of resentment and approval. It

succeeds when it makes resentment and approval subside and
it fails when it produces the equanimity of unknowing."
Visuddhimagga IX, 96

In *A Treatise on the Paramis* by Acariya Dhammapala, translated by Bhikkhu Bodhi, according to the Noble Truths, equanimity's function is "To see things impartially; its manifestation is the subsiding of attraction and repulsion." Its aim is to reflect on beings inheriting the results of their karma. When I sat in Vipassana meditation (see MEDITATION) for 10 days, I experienced a state of equanimity, understanding we are all one and life is to be met with calmness of mind and loving detachment. This profound experience remains with me and was a difficult yet rewarding experience.

Equanimity is included in Buddhism's Seven Factors of Enlightenment. These 7 factors are: Mindfulness (sati), Investigation (shamma vicaya) of the Dhamma; Energy (viriya); Joy (pīti) or Rapture; Relaxation or tranquility (passaddhi) of body and mind; Concentration (samādhi) and Equanimity (upekkha) or to face life with calmness of mind and tranquility, with detachment and without disturbance.

When mind goes back and forth and is full of negativity, worry and judgment and doubt, equanimity is difficult. Equanimity is easier with a calm mind, a heart full of love and compassion for self and others. What is the greatest equanimity? Sylvia Boorstein stated "The ability to feel and understand, in wisdom, that everyone and everything is different, legitimately, as a result of different causes. To live in a friendly, non-adversarial relationship with all things, with all people, and with our lives is the source of greatest equanimity."

EVOLUTION

"When you resolve to evolve, your problems dissolve."
Rev. Michael B. Beckwith,
founder of AGAPE International Spiritual Center in Los Angeles

Michael B. Beckwith stated it perfectly mentioning you must continue to evolve, in mind, body and spirit. Daily, you have 24 hours or 86,400 seconds. This translates to 8,766 hours/year or 31,556,926 seconds/year.

Think about all you can accomplish during that time. Problems dissolve when you acknowledge them and find a solution. That solution is your evolution. As Einstein said, "We can't solve problems by using the same kind of thinking we used when we created them." Choose to evolve. As you evolve, you attune to a higher frequency and awareness.

EXPECTATION

"Expect your every need to be met, expect the answer to every problem, expect abundance on every level and expect to grow spiritually."
Eileen Caddy

In Raymond Holliwell's book, *Working With the Law,* Holliwell spoke about interest and desire forming the backbone to the Law of Attraction or the Law of Vibration, as Bob Proctor calls it. Holliwell stated, "Desire without expectation is ideal wishing." Expect the best and desire the best, believing you will receive it.

Invitation to expand:
What do you expect? Is it the worst or the best? Do you believe you are worthy of receiving the best- what is for your highest good? Do you desire, expect and believe you will receive what you seek? Asking, while expecting it and taking action, are keys to its fruition. If one element is missing, it may remain dormant or take longer to manifest.

FAITH

"Take the first step in faith. You don't have to see the whole staircase, just take the first step."
Martin Luther King, Jr.

In *Think and Grow Rich,* Napoleon Hill stated "Faith is a state of mind that may be induced or created, by affirmation or repeated instructions to the subconscious mind, through the principle of autosuggestion." How do you build your faith? How do you reaffirm the good in your life? Bob Proctor reminds you that "Thoughts become things. If you see it in your mind, you will hold it in your hand." Have faith; believe it to be true and it will be. When a thought arises that doesn't serve you, acknowledge it and say 'Next' until a positive, life affirming thought pops up.

FAMILY/FRIENDS/GRANDPARENTS

"When a child grows up and becomes independent, it opens the doorway for the second cutting of the umbilical cord. In so many cases the family falls from grace, is forced to grow, then reconciles. This is a pattern I see all over the world. This is part of the child's gift giving to the family."
Sobonfu E. Somé

How often have you sat to observe a child for 1 hour watching everything he/she does and says? As an aunt to 3 nieces and 4 nephews, I am continuously blessed with this. Each time is unlike the last as it is fresh and new. Brasilian spiritual healer Ruben Faria stated "Kids have compassion and love without limit-this is pure spirit, very different from material compassion, material love." Kids are open, they have not shut down their intuition. When they hold your hand, they put all of themselves in that experience. Kids are a beautiful example of living in the now.

In his book, *The Breakthrough Experience*, Dr. John F. Demartini describes the mind of kids: "They (children) may have little bodies but they have miraculous and possibly ancient minds. The wisdom is in them and it's in us. All we must do is recognize it." You are all spirits, born tiny and helpless yet brilliant. You can teach a child 11 languages if you wish and he/she will retain them. Napoleon Hill reminds you to "Cherish your visions and your dreams as they are the children of your soul."

Grandparents are special people. They help transport knowledge and wisdom that books cannot. My connection was stronger with my grandmothers. They have a presence that is warm, welcoming and profound. Their stories and recipes move you to a simpler time, to a way of living many young ones have forgotten. Although my grandmothers made the transition, their smiles, stories and hearts are always with me, intertwined in the cells of my soul. They keep me humble and cognizant of who I am, of my lineage, birth and death. What importance do your grandparents have? How do you honor them?

Invitation to expand:

Following the shooting of 7 employees over $2,400 (5 of whom died), author, speaker, coach and former police officer, Orrin Hudson, founded a crime prevention organization entitled Be Someone. He and his team empower children by teaching them chess and how to use their minds to control their life.

When I met and spoke with Orrin, he stated the new currency is KASH which stands for Knowledge, Attitude, Skills and Habits. He teaches young people to "Think it out, don't shoot it out." His goal is to get people to donate $50/month so he can do this important work. If this resonates with you, kindly see www.besomeone.org or contact 770.465.6445. You can help change the world one move at a time.

FEARLESSNESS

**"You can conquer any fear if you will make up your mind to do so.
For remember, fear doesn't exist anywhere except in the mind."**
Dale Carnegie

Fear, like many things is an illusion. It is created in your mind, although not all people live in fear. According to Neale Donald Walsch, in *Conversations With God, Book I,* "Fear is worry magnified. Worry, hate, fear, together with their offshoots: anxiety, bitterness, impatience, unkindness, judgment and condemnation, attack the body at the cellular level. It is impossible to have a healthy body under these conditions. "

Don Miguel Ruiz stated "Death is not the biggest fear we have; our biggest fear is taking the risk to be alive-the risk to be alive and express what we really are." To move beyond this unconscious fear you must do the thing you are afraid of. Here, that would be expressing who and what you are.

In *Life Unlocked*, Harvard Medical School assistant clinical psychiatry professor, Srinivasan S. Pillay, MD, discussed 7 lessons to overcome fear. He stated you are "softwired" and your brain responds to new ways of thinking and sets up new pathways. He gives the following 4 psychological and neurobiological reasons why your brain becomes inflexible: 1) Human drive for love. 2) Desire for permanence. 3) Repetition compulsion (Freudian term indicating adults repeat traumatic experiences) and 4) Delusion of omnipotence (belief in power to do anything).

Also, Dr. Pillay stated that trauma, excessive worry, dread, prejudice and a caged heart may all contribute to fear. To change the conditioned response of fear, new learning (repetition to enhance long term memory) must occur to stimulate new neurons and overwrite old programming or paradigms. Dr. Pillay also suggests using the MAP-Change Approach which stands for Meditation, Attention and Psychological Tools. Attention includes focusing on something other than fear. Psychological tools include asking if you use "genes" or "habit" as excuses and other tools specific to each fear.

Gina Pearson stated "Don't let fear become your friend, for fear will only sabotage your life." Fear has a low frequency and it will drag you down. Oftentimes it contributes to chaos and disease. Remember you attract the frequency you vibrate at (see FREQUENCY). Don't allow it to enter your life. As William Burnham said "The most drastic and usually the most effective remedy for fear is direct action."

FEELINGS

"Feelings are your GPS for life."
Oprah

In *Conversations With God, Book I*, Neal Donald Walsch stated: "Feeling is the language of the soul. If you want to know what's true for you about something, look to how you're feeling about it. Feelings are sometimes difficult to discover and often more difficult to acknowledge. Yet hidden in your deepest feelings is your highest truth. The trick is to get to those feelings."

Osho, in the book *Emotional Wellness*, stated "Feelings cannot be expressed the way thoughts can. Language is created by thought, for thoughts." He mentioned you should not be concerned if you have trouble expressing feelings, be who you are- yourself. Also, men and women differ in their inner core. In general, women intuitively know when people talk and their hearts are not in it. Generally, men, because of conditioning, operate more from their mind or logic. Osho stated that if you are going inward, "The heart is the shortcut to being and the mind is the longest way you can think of." He encourages men to become more heartful and women to be more aware of the logical side of the brain.

FOCUSED ATTENTION

"The number one Life Mastery skill is the development of your capacity to "notice what you are noticing." You direct the Power of Creation with your attention. As you learn to direct your attention, you will find an immense portal of power. It is with your focused attention that you can design, align with and allow the life you truly love and the one that makes the greatest contribution. For this you came."
Mary Morrissey

Dr. Deepak Chopra shared, "Love is attention without judgment. In its natural state, attention only appreciates." Think about a time when you were engulfed in the experience of love and what you were doing or seeing. Time simply melts away in that moment. Athletes refer to this as being in the zone. Others say you are in the 'flow'. All are examples of focused attention. Mihaly Csikszentmihalyi stated when you experience the 'flow,' "You know that what you need to do is possible to do, even though difficult, and sense of time disappears. You forget yourself. You feel part of something larger."

FORGIVENESS

"Forgiveness is born of increased awareness. The more you can see, the easier it is to forgive."
Deepak Chopra, MD

The first person to forgive is you. Once this is accomplished, anyone and everyone else is easy to forgive as they are reflections of you.

How might you forgive yourself? You can begin by giving thanks for everything in your life and focusing on the good. You can affirm "I forgive myself" daily, whenever you feel unworthy, guilty or any negative emotion. Say this aloud as many times as you need to believe it. Once you believe it, your cells and body believe it and life changes. Your energy vibrates at a higher frequency and relationships transform. It transformed my life and I wish it occurs in your life quickly. Do not allow one more day to pass when you do not forgive. Forgive and continue forgiving all the time. Although it is tough, once done, it liberates you and your life.

FRAGRANCE

When I was studying for my Masters in Acupuncture, we were not allowed to use fragrances. Why would that be? According to The Environmental Health Coalition of Western Massachusetts, fragrances have hidden dangers. The chemical and fragrance manufacturers are not mandated to disclose all ingredients. Some fragrances consist of hundreds of chemicals.

According to The Fragranced Products Information Network, FPIN, www.fpinva.org, sales of fragrance materials and chemicals doubled in the 1980s. The FPIN mentioned that with increased usage, asthma, migraines, allergy complaints also increased. Synthetic musk products are in rivers and streams and air quality is also impacted.

According to the Environmental Health Network, www.ehnca.org, hidden dangers of using fragrances or inhaling them (even if you do not use them) include: fatigue; coughing; difficulty breathing; asthma; eye irritation; skin problems; kidney and liver damage. Nausea, vomiting and abdominal pain and various effects on brain and nervous system including headaches, dizziness, depression and irritability may also occur.

Invitation to expand:
Fragrances are found in many things such as air fresheners, household products (fabric softeners, laundry detergent, bleach, etc.); building materials and personal care products including makeup, soap and deodorant. Also, be

aware that natural does not always mean no fragrance as unlisted masking fragrances may be included. Look for 100% fragrance free and read the labels.

Experiment by eliminating fragrant products and reintroducing them. Notice how you feel and do not be afraid to make another person aware of your sensitivity to his/her fragrance. As a chemically sensitive human, I find essential oils work beautifully without harmful side effects. Visit www.pagona.com for more information about these gems.

FREEDOM

"If there be a human being who is freer than I, then I shall necessarily become his slave. If I am freer than any other, then he will become my slave. Therefore equality is an absolutely necessary condition of freedom."
Mikhail A. Bakunin, Russian revolutionist 1814-1876

When you think of being free, many situations may come to mind. Perhaps you think 'If this job wasn't costing me 50 hours of my time/week I'd be free' or 'If my mom or dad wasn't telling me how to do what I do, I'd be free' or 'When I make a million dollars I'll be free.' Freedom is much more than these scenarios. My definition of freedom is "Freedom= infinite abundance + choice + love + truth." With choice, you have abundance and with abundance and choice, you fly with wings that live in truth and love.

Invitation to expand:
Mary Morrissey stated "Problems are really opportunities to liberate and experience freedom." What if you weekly reflect on Mary's quote to see what wisdom lies in your problems? What if you also ask Barbara De Angelis' question, "What do I need to let go of to be free?" What does FREEDOM look like for YOU?

Wendell Willkie said it well with the words "Freedom is an indivisible word. If we want to enjoy it and fight for it, we must be prepared to extend it to everyone, whether they are rich or poor, whether they agree with us or not, no matter what their race or the color of their skin."

GENES

"The language of the genes has a simple alphabet, not with twenty-six letters but four. These are four different DNA bases—adenine, guanine, cytosine and thymine (A, G, C and T for short). The bases are arranged in words of three letters such as CGA or TGG. Most of the words code for different amino acids joined together to make proteins, the building blocks of the body."
John Stephen Jones, *The Language of the Genes:*
Biology, History and the Evolutionary Future

According to Dean Ornish, MD Founder of the Preventive Medicine Research Institute and author of *The Spectrum*, "Our latest studies show that when you change your lifestyle, you change your genes-turning on genes that prevent disease and turning off genes that cause prostate cancer, breast cancer, heart disease and other illnesses- over 500 genes in only 3 months." Did you know this? Do you understand the powerful implications of your lifestyle?

GROWTH

"Growth is the willingness to let reality be new every moment."
Deepak Chopra, MD

Pearl S. Buck reminds you that "Love dies when growth stops." Daily you have a choice to continue learning, applying and growing or to stand still, absorbing negativity. You are a product of your family and environment and for growth to occur, changes to that environment may be made. Whatever situation you are in, YOU are in charge of your growth. YOU have the daily choice to move forward or backward.

Bob Proctor shared that "The only thing that can grow is the thing you give energy to." It is the application of clarity, choice, discernment, integrity, love, knowledge and wisdom that promotes growth. What choice will you make- to grow or not to grow? What will you give energy to?

GOALS

Bob Proctor expressed, **"Your real purpose in life is to develop yourself. To successfully do this you must always be working toward a goal."**

Napoleon Hill stated that "A goal is a dream with a deadline." What you desire is first noticed and with that acknowledgment, a plan outlined to develop that desire. This plan has a timeframe, or as Hill states, a deadline. Often you may not know when success will be reached yet you can measure whether you reached your goals.

According to Gene Donohue, founder of Top Achievement, goals must be **SMART**- **S**pecific, **M**easurable, **A**ttainable, **R**ealistic and **T**imely. To be specific, goals must answer the 6 "W" – Who, What, Where, When, Which and Why. An example of a specific goal is 'I swim for 30 minutes 5 days/week.' To be measurable, you answer 'How will you know when this goal is accomplished'? An attainable goal is one you are willing and able to work towards. A timely goal has a deadline, otherwise there is no urgency. Bob Proctor also stated, "You must have a goal more powerful than your paradigm." (See Paradigms)

Bob Proctor makes a great distinction between purpose, vision and goals stating, "Your purpose explains what you are doing with your life. Your vision explains how you are living your purpose. Your goals enable you to realize your vision."

Invitation to expand:

Take Bob Proctor's quote about purpose, vision and goals and apply it to your life. What are you doing with your life (purpose)? How are you living your purpose (your vision)? What goals did you set (realize your vision)?

GRATITUDE

"Whenever you are facing any form of resistance, gratitude has the power to quickly dissolve it. This is true whether the hindrance comes from inside of you or outside of you."
Peggy McColl

Gratitude and trust are ingredients I do not leave home without. They help me in countless situations including travel. I travel safely, remaining open and grateful for surprises, serendipity and whomever and whatever is to appear. (Years ago, a friend's husband suggested I write a book about these often surprising and unbelievable travel adventures. Perhaps this will be a future endeavor).

As a volunteer acupuncture trainer for the Pan African Acupuncture Project (PAAP), www.panafricanacupuncture.com, I was humbled, honored and grateful for the beautiful souls I trained, treated and witnessed in one of the poorest countries in Sub Saharan Africa- Uganda. Before returning to the states, I arrived in Ethiopia without any contacts and fluency in Aramaic or Ethiopian languages. My native Greek could not help.

At the airport, I gave thanks for meeting an Ethiopian travel buddy, trusting he/she would appear when appropriate. Shortly afterwards, I heard an English speaking man talking with a group of young people. We spoke and he gave me the number of a man who became a friend. Thank you Siltan, for the day you showed me your beautiful country. Your generosity of spirit, time and energy are blessings that remain with me. Holding the frequency of gratitude as often as possible will transform situations and your life. People appear, things previously unavailable become available, a new reality opens up. My life is infused with hundreds of these magical events. As I write this, a huge smile permeates as I recall the latest one beautifully unfolding in my life...

In *The Answer is You* PBS special, Rev. Michael B. Beckwith described 3 stages of giving gratitude and thanksgiving. They are: "1) Be grateful for EVERYTHING 2) Be grateful for the seeming negativity. 3) Be grateful for being ALIVE, period. Unattached to anything." He stated that if you are the same person 365 days/yr. you went backwards. The Universe you live in is progressive. The 'negative' comes into your life to help you grow. He continued stating, "Go on a hunt for what you can be grateful for."

Mike Dooley, author of *Infinite Possibilities* shares, "Give thanks and praise to LIFE, its grace and its unfailing principles for having already manifested your dreams." The act of giving thanks and staying in a grateful vibration, frees your mind from worry and helps attract more things to be grateful for. It is also a scientific fact that gratitude and appreciation affect your health, intelligence, creativity and problem solving. Psychotherapist and sound healer, Tom Kenyon stated "When you make a change in your emotional state, you change the biochemistry of your brain and the functioning of your physiology."

Invitation to expand:
What if you did as Rev. Michael B. Beckwith suggested and look for what you can be grateful for instead of what you can complain about? How would your day change? What if you woke up to gratitude and fell asleep to gratitude? Try it and share what transpires.

GRIEF/SADNESS

"Tears are the river of life washing away the old to make way for something new."
Shakti Gawain, author of *The Four Levels of Healing*

When understanding and grieving a loss, Guy Finley states that through a beloved's loss the following awareness occurs "Part of the pain of a loss is losing a way we knew ourselves -- through someone else. The true student of life -- who loves the Divine -- must be willing to see that when God takes from us the temporary forms he does including those we love, he simultaneously offers us the possibility of understanding that much suffering occurred because we mistook what passed for something everlasting."

Finley shared that when you understand that Only God, Love, and the Light of Truth -- call it what you will -- is eternal, "Your battle to learn this truth frees you from what appears to be a loss." Continue growing and expanding and the energy of your loss will diminish. It will be transmuted into joy and life again as the person may have left your physical world yet the energy of that person always remains.

HABITS PRODUCE REALITY

"You and I are the product of someone else's habitual thinking."
Bob Proctor

To be highly effective, it is important to follow certain habits. In *The 7 Habits of Highly Effective People*, Stephen Covey described the following 7 Habits: 1) Be proactive 2) Begin with the end in mind 3) Put first things first 4) Think win/win 5) Seek first to understand then to be understood 6) Synergize and 7) Sharpen the Saw.

I discuss each habit further and encourage you to read and study Covey's book.

Habit 1, being proactive entails taking responsibility and initiative for your life to make things happen. Habits of highly proactive people include not placing blame (reactive). Instead, they respond in alignment with their values; exercising conscious choice while applying proactive language on things they can do something about. Examples of proactive language include "I choose" instead of the reactive "I can't" and "I prefer" instead of the reactive "I must."

Habit 2, beginning with the end in mind is based on the principle that all things are created twice. First they are created mentally and then physically. An example is building a home. The blueprint is created before the physical building is erected. A great way to begin with the end in mind is to create a mission statement incorporating vision, values, guidance, wisdom and power. There must be involvement to have commitment. Visualizing, affirmations, identifying roles and goals are also used here.

Habit 3, putting first things first involves fulfilling Habits 1 and 2. It involves exercising free will to do what must be done. To accomplish: place to do items in 4 quadrants, distinguishing between urgent and important; urgent and not important; not urgent and important and not urgent and not important. The focus is to fulfill quadrant II- important and not urgent items first.

Habit 4, thinking win/win seeks mutual benefit for all in a cooperative space. Both solutions mutually satisfy and benefit. This is based on plenty for everyone and involves the following five dimensions: character (integrity, maturity, abundance mentality); relationships; agreements; systems and processes.

Habit 5 involves seeking first to understand then be understood. This includes empathic listening, or listening to understand, not to reply. Another way of stating it is to diagnose before you prescribe.

Habit 6, synergizing allows your heart and mind to remain open to new possibilities. Valuing differences is essential as well as believing in a better option while operating from a place of excitement, security and adventure.

Lastly, **Habit 7**, sharpen the saw allows the previous habits to manifest. It entails balanced self-renewal. It renews the four dimensions- mental, physical, spiritual and social/emotional.

Stephen R. Covey concluded with "Achieving unity-oneness-with ourselves, with our loved ones, with our friends and working associates is the highest and best and most delicious fruit of the Seven Habits." My hope is that you implement the 7 Habits into your life and celebrate the profound changes.

WHAT DOES HAPPINESS MEAN TO YOU?

Jonathan C Cordeiro, Jccimagineer, Purist, Human:
"Happiness is love. Happiness is accomplishment. It is turning a negative into a positive. Happiness is being able to accept this moment and realize that whether it is easy, difficult, good, bad, short or long, it is my moment now. Happiness is knowing that although the glass is half empty, it is half full and I can drink. Happiness is being aware that I choose to be happy, although society might not understand how I can be. "When life gives you lemons-make lemonade"... If you like raspberries or more sugar or iced tea, make a raspberry flavored Arnold Palmer. It is your glass to drink. Happiness is that feeling in your gut that makes you realize you are on the right path. It is your internal sensor. Whatever makes you feel happy and aware, continue to feel it."

Ana-Laura, age 11:
"I think that happiness is having fun and getting lost in your imagination. It can also be peaceful, like when you read a good book or watch a good movie and be with the people of your imagination or play with your pet.

If you are happy, you help and do stuff for friends and family but you also don't have to do anything you don't want to. Happiness is when you are with friends and family and surrounded by people who care about you. If you are happy, you don't lie and you aren't anybody else but you. You don't carry the weight of trying to pretend. Happiness is what you want it to be."

Meredith Evangelisti, Bikram yoga teacher, co-founder www.hotdropapparel.com:
"Happiness is knowing that I do something that I love, teaching yoga, and that it makes a difference to the people around me. I feel I am teaching others to find the way to good health which will result in happiness."

Mike D. Joseph, college student, age 21:
"Being at peace, not necessarily being at peace with the world but being at peace with yourself. Being happy is not for the moment; a thrill is being happy for the moment but true happiness is being happy for a lifetime."

Ellie Hwong, From Sabah, Malaysia, Practitioner of Nichiren Daishonin's Buddhism (Soka Gakkai):

"Happiness means being present at this moment. It means making a conscious decision to be happy no matter what happens. It means being appreciative of people around you, especially family and loved ones. Nothing stays permanent, everything changes. Sadness won't last forever and temporary happiness will soon fade as well. You will never be as young as you are today. The greatest happiness is to live with no regret. People who complain are never satisfied and never happy. Instead take action and make a positive change. Be courageous! I dare you to be happy. "

Kahuna Kalei'iliahi:
"Happiness is also a state of mind and consciousness that involves the awareness that we are all connected to everything and everyone, including God. It is a high harmonious state of mind where the Human is in tune with their own Divinity and connected to that Source which is where true happiness comes from...inside. As a result, we can access it anytime through the conscious connections with our minds and hearts to the Source, which is in our hearts. True happiness is not dependent on outside things but rather an

inner contentment and comes to the Human that can say "It is well with my Soul," no matter what is happening in and outside of them."

Harry Kasparian, psychologist:
"Happiness is the state of mind predicated by a healthy soul, mind, body and heart which promote insatiable desire to learn and serve humanity with passion and compassion."

Richard Mandell, L. Ac., Founder/Executive Director of The Pan African Acupuncture Project (PAAP), www.panafricanacupuncture.org:
"Happiness is the ability to give and receive love, to be loving and being loved. Similar to health, it embraces the interconnectedness of everything, it dismisses being judgmental and thrives on seeing the uniqueness, the specialness in each of us."

Tofoul Marzouki:
"Happiness is when my body and mind release positive energy, a kind of energy that makes me feel it's not bad being here and constrained, trapped in this watery flesh. Happiness is when you know and feel that you gain pleasure from all you know and have. True happiness comes with inspiration and is significant when it is shared. When you stop trying to prove yourself that is when you have inner happiness. Real happiness should not be expressed; it is only felt and sensed. It should not be condemned, praised nor analyzed. Happiness can be portrayed but there is no point if it is not genuinely recognized by the self."

Alexandra Mattioli, niece, age 7:
"Happiness means love. When you give popsicles to people. Flowers."

Dr. Tanya Miszko Kefer, Ed.D., L.Ac., Exercise Physiologist, Acupuncturist, owner www.prescriptivehealth.com:

"Happiness is a sense of peace with who you are and where you are in life; a feeling of lightness yet full of life."

Leszek Mularski:
"Who are You happiness? Do I know You?

How I can be happy if I know people are dying from hunger and kids are killed, is it possible to be happy?

Yes I remember You" happiness" such a selfish feeling.

I was happy standing on snowy peaks, looking around and falling in love with nature's beauty.

Could happiness be such a trivial feeling? No it cannot be.

I can get help from mentors like Socrates, Platoon and Kierkegaard.

Did Socrates say happiness is impossible to reach?

Did Kierkegaard say "There isn't objective reality so happiness couldn't be real?"

I think happiness is a different feeling for everybody. For me, it means "winning" and eureka. I have this light which makes me happy. "All is form" but creative form is immortal and makes me happy."

Stathi Nikolaidis, Athens, Greece:
"Happiness is a state of well-being that includes positive emotions. Where is joy and why are many unhappy? Humans were created to be happy but our perfect creator gave us the free will to experience the opposite of happiness.

Happiness comes from looking outside the box, remaining as objective as possible and honoring the advice I give others. It also includes sharing with loved ones and laughing a lot. While some may call me a romantic fool, I am happy knowing I make others happy."

David Roe, Master Mind friend:
"Happiness is stopping long enough to take an INTERNAL stock take of all the things that make you smile and then, in moments of calmness, taking time to give gratitude for each of these blessings."

Sandra Roe, Master Mind friend:
"Happiness is the awareness of the beauty that is within that brings forth a feeling of gratitude and understanding of the magnificence of life."

Retired nurse, age 82:

"Happiness is a feeling of contentment; feeling fortunate that I accomplished and fulfilled a purpose in life. I am happy I have the same set of friends for 60 years. I especially am happy when I am able to do things for those less fortunate, in deeds, words and actions. That gives me a great sense of happiness and fulfillment."

Errol Stephenson:
"Happiness is hearing that song."

Cianna Tangishaka, age 8:
"Happiness means when I am happy that everyone around me is happy. It is also when I am proud of myself because I made my goals."

Afia Yeboah, case manager, age 25:
"Happiness to me means knowing God. He is the author and finisher of my faith. I know when I have him all things work out for my good."

Dr. Leticia Vargas, OB/GYN:
"Happiness...is being in tune with your inner spirit and being in peace with yourself and where you are in life."

Eleni Vogiatzis, niece, age 13:
"Happiness means dreaming as big as the ocean."

WHAT is happiness?

"If I wait to be happy, I'll wait forever. If I choose to be happy now, I'll be happy forever."
Unknown

In 1965, George Romney wrote *Success, The Pursuit of The Difficult.* His first paragraph reads: "Happiness is never the result-it is a byproduct-it comes from something else: from service, from the pursuit of a goal larger than yourself, from the pursuit, of difficult, which makes people strong, rather than from the pursuit of easy things, which makes people weak."

Thich Nhat Hanh shared, "The amount of happiness that you have depends on the amount of freedom you have in your heart." Thus, a heart with more freedom would be happier. His Holiness the Karmapa shared, "Sometimes we develop grand concepts of what happiness might look like for us, but if we pay attention, we can see that there are little symbols of happiness in every breath that we take."

As glimpsed from the above responses and the young and older people interviewed, people's perception of happiness varies. For some, happiness means a response to pleasure. However, for many, it comes from within or from helping others. According to Michio Kushi, author of The *Book of Macrobiotics* "Joyous life is a natural result of health and it gives joy and happiness to people surrounding us, like the sun which radiates its light and warmth to every life upon earth..."

In his book, *The Path to Love*, Dr. Deepak Chopra stated that in polls, when people were asked if they are happy, about 70% said yes. This was consistent globally, across age groups from young to old. The one exception was the very poor who seem to be less happy.

Imagine a country's success determined by something other than the GDP (Gross Domestic Product). In the South Asian country of Bhutan, success is evaluated by the GNH (Gross National Happiness) of its people. Under GNH, everyone aspires to live a meaningful, happy life. Happiness links Bhutan's people to the success of its economy. Bhutan invests in 75% of its land (agriculture, hills and mountains). This creates local jobs and encourages tourism while increasing wealth and happiness.

WHAT DOES HEALTH MEAN TO YOU?

Randy B., EMT, age 26:
"To be healthy means to have a good constitution; to be resilient and have longevity. It also means to be a human white blood cell, progressive and prosperous with the teachings of God. "

Dora, translator, age 53:
"Health means time and hope. It is being able to live long enough to see

my daughter get married and hold my grandkids. Health is taking care of the body I inhabit: my legs to go places and my arms and hands to hug someone and work. Health means caring for my mind and spirit so I can appreciate life more. Life can end in a second; it is difficult to keep this in mind. I hope to have the healthy body and soul to enjoy life while it lasts."

Meredith Evangelisti, Bikram Yoga teacher, co-founder of www. hotdropapparel.com:
"Health and happiness are both very important to me. I couldn't have one without the other and it is hard for me to see where one ends and the other begins. Being healthy means living an active lifestyle and eating well and also having a sound, happy mind. Before practicing Bikram yoga, I lived an active lifestyle and ate healthy foods but my mind was all over the place. Bikram yoga helped me gain control over my emotions and my mind in even the most stressful situations."

Harry Kasparian, psychologist:
"Health is the ingestation and assimilation of tangible and intangible health promoting and sustaining ingredients for spiritual, physical, mental and emotional aspects of my life."

Richard Mandell, L.Ac., PAAP Founder/Executive Director, www. panafricanacupuncture.org:
"Health is a reflection of one's relationship--to oneself and to others, to one's internal and external environment. It is the knowledge and the acceptance of the interconnectedness of all things."

Tofoul Marzouki:
"Health is something I long for when I'm ill and could be taken for granted, positively and negatively. Health can be affected by exterior elements but is also a state of mind. Over obsessing about health is unhealthy. It is a crucial matter for me when I need to regain it. When health is threatened, I make adjustments. I am not health conscious nor do I believe in prevention or health plans. My mental health is my priority and then my body follows. For example, I exercise to feel happy and enjoy myself, not because it is good for my body."

Dr. Tanya Miszko Kefer, Ed.D., L.Ac., Exercise Physiologist, Acupuncturist, owner of www.prescriptivehealth.com:

"Health is an overall term that encompasses your whole being; spirit, mind and body. To me, health is balance in your day, a solid spiritual practice, an invigorating exercise program, clean living, a sound mind and an appetite for knowledge."

Leslaw Mularski:

"Health means to live life to the fullest according to my age and limits. It means to live life without any help from medicine like flu shots, vitamins and antibiotics."

Stathi Nikolaidis, Athens, Greece:

"For me, health corresponds with society's view of it. To have a healthy crowd is to have to a well- informed crowd that is given the truth about everything including all knowledge about disease and prevention. The knowledge exists for us to be healthy and strong but we are not. We rely heavily on medications instead of prevention and natural interventions. Being healthy means decreased stress, breathing clean air and eating clean, nutritious food. It means finding the power within to heal ourselves."

Retired nurse, age 82:

"As an octogenarian, health to me is not having any severe or mental illness, just minor aches and pains. I haven't had a cold in 50 years. I have always been able to function. I consider that a blessing."

David Roe, Master Mind friend:

"Health is achieved by believing that the essence of our being is perfection and that the core of our foundation is balanced and at ease.

Our lack of faith in this fact causes us to be imbalanced in our thinking-not at ease or "diseased" and this is the cause of health issues. To have health, we must gain greater awareness of the truth of our being. From this understanding we will process disease from our thinking and the result will be health in all respects."

Sandra Roe, Master Mind friend:
"Health is choosing to create balance in all aspects of our life and becoming aware of the perfection in everything."

Christine Tangishaka:
"Total health, is a state of being aware and accepting (or working on) all aspects of one's current existence; physical, emotional, spiritual and psychological. Each contributes greatly to the whole as you cannot be fully healthy with unattended gaping deficits in one area."

Dr. Leticia Vargas, OB/GYN:
"Health means to be balanced. Mind, body, spirit connection in sync. I tell my patients to be healthy they have to sleep at least 8 hours each night; eat healthfully and mindfully; exercise daily; de-stress daily and detox regularly."

Afia Yeboah, case manager, age 25:
"Good health to me means having peace of mind. "

Lao Tzu, author of Tao Te Ching, translated by John C. H Wu
offers the following health wisdom:
"To realize that our knowledge is ignorance,
This is a noble insight.
To regard our ignorance as knowledge,
This is a mental sickness.
Only when we are sick of our sickness
Shall we cease to be sick.
The Sage is not sick, for being sick of sickness;
This is the secret of health."

"Every human being is the author of his own health or disease."
Hindu Prince Gautama Siddhartha, Buddhism founder, 563-483 B.C

According to Maoshing Ni, PhD's translation of the NEIJING SUWEN, or The Yellow Emperor's Classic of Medicine, preface XIII, health is defined as "Health and well-being can be achieved only by remaining centered in spirit, guarding against the squandering of energy, promoting the constant flow of qi and blood, maintaining hormonal balance of yin and yang, adapting to the changing seasonal and yearly macrocosmic influences and nourishing one's self preventively. This is the way to a long and happy life."

Brené Brown shared, "We are the most in-debt, obese, addicted and medicated adult cohort in U.S. history." Upon reviewing Brené Brown's words, there is much truth to her words. How do you change to become less in debt, addicted and medicated? Thomas Edison suggested one way with the following words "The doctor of the future will give no medicine but will interest his patient in the care of the human frame, in diet and in the cause and prevention of disease." In America, prevention is, unfortunately, not given much attention. In Europe and Asia, preventative measures are embraced quicker than in the states. Simplifying your life and living within your means may change many things including the health of your body, mind and bank account. Rachel Naomi offers another insight stating "Healing may not be so much about getting better as about letting go of everything that isn't you-all of the expectations, all of the beliefs and becoming who you are."

In *As A Man Thinketh*, James Allen stated "If you would perfect your body, guard your mind. If you would renew your body, renew your mind." Everything is made up of energy. Thus, food, like thoughts is made up of energy that depletes or energy that nourishes. If you nourish yourself with life promoting food and life promoting thoughts, your life may be happier than one who eats processed food and constantly digests anger and sadness.

Allen also mentioned "Change of diet will not help a man who will not change his thoughts." If you constantly remain in anger, negativity and bitterness, you may hinder the absorption of food. You can eat the purest, freshest, most alive food yet think the worst thoughts and thus, the low vibrational thoughts will become a part of the food. Dr. Yeshe Donden, Dalai Lama's physician stated it well with "Health is the proper relationship between microcosm, which is man and the macrocosm, which is the universe. Disease is a disruption of this relationship."

HUGS

"Oxytocin connects us to other people; oxytocin makes us feel

what other people feel. It's easy to cause people's brains to release oxytocin. Let me show you. Come here. Give me a hug."

Paul Zak

In The *Hug Therapy Book*, Kathleen Keating, R.N, MA shared, "Hug therapy is the practice of administering hugs for the sole purpose of curing and healing or of preserving health. Hug therapy is not free. The cost is the strength it requires to be vulnerable. The fee for hugging is the risk that our hugs will be rebuffed or misinterpreted." She mentioned many hug types including: bear hugs, frame hugs, cheek hugs, side to side hugs and heart centered hugging.

Paul Zak shared "[You need] eight hugs a day. You'll be happier and the world will be a better place." Imagine 8 hugs a day from loved ones! While working in the ER as a cardiac research technician, I had the opportunity to watch many procedures. The day after watching open heart surgery, I visited the patient whose heart I saw. He held a stuffed animal close to his chest and spoke about what brought him to this stage in life.

What benefit would he receive by hugging a teddy bear daily? Hugs are very therapeutic and as Paul Zak mentioned, your brain releases oxytocin making you feel connected. Kathleen Keating stated "Hugging affirms physical being; builds self-esteem; fosters altruism and eases tension." I offer you an abundance of hugs!!

HUMAN HEART

"If you are identified with the heart, then your desires will be of a still higher nature, higher than the mind. You will become more aesthetic, more sensitive, more alert, more loving."
Osho

In *Fractal Time: The Secret of 2012 and a New World Age*, Gregg Braden stated, "The human heart generates the strongest magnetic field in the body, nearly 5,000 times stronger than that of the brain. This field creates a doughnut shaped pattern that extends beyond the physical body and was measured at distances five to eight feet from the physical heart."

What is the implication of this? The emotions you create in your life, namely, positive emotions, increase the hormonal balance and heart rhythm and thus the heart's magnetic field responds. Institute of HeartMath studies, (www.prwebdirect.com/releases/2008/10/prweb1415844.htm) found that negative emotions may affect 1,400 biochemical body changes including poor performance, hormonal imbalance and mental fogginess.

IDEAS

"An idea manifests through the physical body. It alters the vibration causing change in behavior."
Bob Proctor

It takes one good idea to change your life. Bob Proctor mentions that "Words=dressed up ideas." When you read a book, it is also many ideas or a picture painted in words. Dr. John Murray states "We are according to our system of ideas." When you receive ideas, write them down. Always keep an idea journal with you, ready to hold any idea that enters your mind. Ideas, like everything, consist of energy. One idea may change your life. It changed the Wright Brothers and Edison's lives and many others. Stay open to any and all ideas, for you never know when you may allow one to use you and in so doing, transform you and thousands of others. This book was once an idea written in my idea book years ago. It is now reality, thanks to the many who believed in me.

Invitation to expand:
In the film *Inception*, one of the main characters stated, "An idea is like a virus- resilient and highly contagious. Smallest seed of an idea can grow. It can grow to define or destroy you." What are your ideas? How are they manifesting in your life? Are they destroying or defining you?

IGNORANCE

"Not to know is bad but not to wish to know is worse."
West African proverb

Tom Kenyon stated it well with the following: "Don't condemn a person because their experience is different than yours or their culture is different than yours. Look in the box with curiosity. Oh it's a fellow human being, how did they experience that?" Ignorance is widespread and often undectable as many are unaware of what they do not know.

Confucius reminds you that "Real knowledge is to know the extent of one's ignorance." When you know that you do not know, you are open to learning. However, when you think you know, you are closed off to learning. Stay open, remain inquisitive and live now. Remember Martin Luther King's words "Nothing in the world is more dangerous than sincere ignorance and conscientious stupidity."

IMAGINATION

"Our imagination is the most important faculty we possess. It can be our greatest resource or our most formidable adversary. It is through our imagination that we discern possibilities and options. Imagination is the deepest voice of the soul and can be heard clearly only through cultivation and careful attention. A relationship with our imagination is a relationship with our deepest self."
Pat B. Allen, *Art Is a Way of Knowing*

Albert Einstein stated "Imagination is more important than knowledge." Imagination creates the possibility of any world. As kids, your imagination was free of the conditioning you are exposed to as an adult. In this land of play and pretend, dreams and unlimited possibilities exist. As you become older, you are conditioned to believe imagination is daydreaming and has no place in your life. From imagination, ideas arise and from ideas, choices exist. From choices, possibilities present and new ways of seeing and living are born.

Invitation to expand:
Napoleon Bonaparte said "The human race is governed by its imagination." If you refuse your imagination, you accept a dull life full of less than your greatness. What if, instead, you devoted 10 minutes a day to your imagination? What would that look like?

INCOME

"Only when the last tree has died and the last river has been poisoned and the last fish been caught will we realize we cannot eat money."
Cree Indian Proverb

From what do you receive your income? Do you own a business or work for someone else? Income is a reflection of the amount of service and value you provide. T. Harv Eker, in SpeedWealth stated "You will be paid in direct proportion to the value you deliver according to the marketplace." If you provide service to millions of people, you will make more money than if you serve hundreds of people.

Often people pursue large amounts of income to the detriment of their health, family or relationships. Balance is key and as the Cree Indian Proverb states, money cannot be eaten. Money is very important yet wealth is more than income and assets. It entails an abundance of health; income; freedom; inner peace; harmonious and loving relationships and prosperous and purposeful living. Bob Proctor stated that "Doing a good job is where you get your psychic income from."

Brian Tracy made the following suggestion "Invest three percent of your income in yourself (self-development) in order to guarantee your future." Many schools of thought exist about this. One suggestion is to invest 3% while another may be to invest 10%. Whatever percentage you choose, ensure that it is continuously applied to your self-improvement account and that you consistently invest in yourself. Mary Morrissey reminds you that "The first currency is never money, it is always ideas."

INNER PEACE

Symptoms of Inner Peace by Saskia Davis:
"A tendency to think and act spontaneously instead of acting on fears attached to past experience.
An unmistakable ability to enjoy the moment.
A loss of interest in judging other people.

A loss of interest in interpreting the actions of others.

An inability to worry (this is a very serious symptom).

Frequent overwhelming episodes of appreciation.

Frequent acts of smiling.

An increasing tendency to let things happen instead of making them happen.

An increased susceptibility to the love extended by others as well as the uncontrollable urge to extend it."

How many look for peace outside yourselves only to be disappointed when it doesn't arrive or is short lived? Thich Nhat Hanh reminds you, "Real strength is not in power, money or weapons but in deep, inner peace." When inner peace is applied to humanity, profound changes occur. People become more compassionate and offer their true selves and feelings. The Dalai Lama spoke about this with the words "World peace must develop from inner peace. Peace is not just mere absence of violence. Peace is, I think, the manifestation of human compassion."

INSIGHT

**"Insight enables you to know your own heart,
Clarity enables you to accept without illusions,
Objectivity enables you to view any person or situation with
compassion."**
Deepak Chopra, MD author, *The Path to Love*

Dr. Deepak Chopra also shared, "Real change is accompanied by an insight and "Insights bring truth which is love in action." When you realize change within, your environment and life also change. For this change to occur, new information, ideas or insight is needed. Without insight, the same knowledge circulates which may lead to repeating your actions, in other words, not moving forward. As Dr. Chopra stated, this insight allows more love in your life as truth is seen and spoken.

Thich Nhat Hanh invites you to "Live deeply every moment of life-concentrated." Get insight into yourself and the other person. "Person is not your enemy, person is yourself- person needs you to be transformed."

Invitation to expand: What if you review a month of your life and ask what your insight gave birth to? The insight gave birth to the awareness of _____. What observations might propel you to greater insight?

INSPIRATION

"Don't give up trying to do what you really want to do. Where there is love and inspiration, I don't think you can go wrong."
Ella Fitzgerald

Jack London shared "You can't wait for inspiration. You have to go after it with a club." Actively seek avenues of inspiration. Upon examining the word, inspiration, you find in and spirit. People living inspirational lives are in a state of communing with a Divine presence, Spirit or whatever you wish to call it. Many artists, composers, musicians all become one with their creation, some unaware of how their talent is expressed. One sister, Pascalia, shared that when she creates her art, while physically in her body, she is transported to another space full of ideas expressed in color and form. It is from this place of inspiration that she creates beautiful and bold abstract art.

Invitation to expand:
What inspires you to live an authentic, compassion, creative life? How do you access that inspiration? What can you do today to create more opportunities for breathing that in, with each step you take, each word you speak and each action you perform?

INTEGRITY

"More than any other trait, the presence of absence of honesty, that is integrity, is a window into the soul of another person."
Gordon Livingstone

In Hamlet, a character named Polonius told his son, Laertes: "This above all: to thine own self be true and it must follow, as the night the day, thou cannot be false to any man." When you operate from a place of integrity, much of the power of your "itty bitty shitty committee" is lost. You know where you come from and the journey you travel. You keep your word and it is easy for others to respect and do business with you. They trust you because you trust yourself, operating from honesty. As R. Buckminster Fuller stated "Integrity is the essence of everything successful."

INTUITION

"The Intuitive Mind is a sacred gift and the rational mind is a faithful servant. We have created a society that honors the servant and has forgotten the gift."
Albert Einstein

In his book, *Heaven and Earth*, world renowned spiritual medium, James Van Praagh stated "You must learn to cultivate your mind and intuition, read and study a variety of spiritual philosophies and perhaps even attend classes to rely on your own intuitive ability." How many of you doubt your intuition and believe a certain % of the population is psychic or intuitive? It is true that you are all intuitive yet some developed their intuitive faculties more than others.

As Mary Morrissey states "Intuition points the way yet doesn't tell you why." Should you choose to honor it, it leads you to your truest wisdom, to Divine guidance and your highest self. Your intuition knows more than you do. Trust it and allow it to guide you.

Dr. Richard Bartlett reminds you to "Trust your hunches and intuition- they are closer to reality than your perceived reality as they are based on far more information."

JOURNEY

"The truth is that there is no journey. You are right now what you are attempting to be. You are right now where you are attempting to go."
Conversations with God, Book III by Neale Donald Walsch

Lao Tzu once said "A journey of a thousand miles must begin with a single step." For anything to happen, for example, to open a business, get married or relocate, a first step must be taken. Further action is needed and although you may not know the how of it, that first step is needed.

Great wisdom is found in the words of Greg Anderson "Focus on the journey, not the destination. Joy is found not in finishing an activity but in doing it." In other words, focus on the now, what is present here and give no thought to how you will get to the destination. You are often rewarded with growth that would not have been possible or may have been delayed if the journey was not undertaken.

KARMA

"Things don't arbitrarily happen to you. Events in your business are the reflection of your thoughts, the echo of your own actions and the thinking behind them. In the East, this truth is reflected in the idea of karma and in the West the Golden Rule. The core of the principle is this: You are at cause in your life and in your business."
John Assaraf and Murray Smith, authors of *The Answers*

In *The Power of the Soul,* Dr. Zhi Gang Sha spoke about many things including karma. He stated "Karma is the record of services, divided into good (good services in past lives and this life including love, compassion, honesty and kindness) and bad karma (unpleasant services including harming, taking advantage of, stealing, etc.)."

Dr. Zhi Gang Sha suggested simple practices for increasing good karma by offering unconditional universal service in the form of 7 universal aspects: love; forgiveness; peace; healing; blessing; harmony and enlightenment. Universal love offers love to all souls while universal forgiveness forgives all souls. Universal peace offers peace to all, embracing every country, society, universe, religion and race. For universal harmony, one must be in harmony with all aspects of self, including personal, family, Earth and planetary harmony.

Invitation to expand:

According to Dr. Zhi Gang, if you serve unpleasantly, you learn lessons. However, if you serve well, you receive blessings. You may wish to clear bad karma by first stating Dr. Zhi Gang's mantra below and singing the Soul Song entitled: "Love, Peace and Harmony" as many times as possible. If this resonates with you, I suggest reviewing Dr. Zhi Gang's book, *The Power of The Soul* for more healing practices, suggestions and wisdom.

Mantra:

"Dear soul, mind and body of the Divine Soul Song, "Love, Peace and Harmony" downloading to my soul.

I love you, honor you and appreciate you.

Please heal my ____(make request for physical, emotional, mental, spiritual body).

Please purify my soul, heart, mind and body.

Please clear my bad karma.

Please rejuvenate my soul, heart, mind and body.

Please transform my life, including my relationships and finances.

Please enlighten my soul, heart, mind and body.

I am very grateful.

Thank you."

Soul Song, "Love, Peace and Harmony" (in English and Chinese):

"I love my heart and soul	"Wo ai wo xin he ling
I love all humanity	Wo ai quan ren lei
Join hearts and souls together	Wan ling rong he mu she sheng
Love, peace and harmony	Xiang ai ping an he xie
Love, peace and harmony"	Xiang ai ping an he xie"

KINDNESS

"Kindness in words creates confidence. Kindness in thinking creates profoundness. Kindness in giving creates love."
Lao Tzu

PAGONA

What if our paradigm was to create kindness daily, even offering it to those we think do not deserve it? What would our world look like if this was a foundational premise we operated from?

LAUGHTER

"Everybody laughs the same in every language because laughter is a universal connection."
Yakov Smirnoff

The film *Dr. Patch Adams,* mentioned, "Laughter moves lymph fluid, promotes oxygenation of body cells and organs and improves circulation." Laughter helps relax you. When you laugh, you contract 15 facial muscles and stimulate the zygomatic muscle. Meanwhile, the epiglottis causes the larynx to half close resulting in irregular air intake, making you gasp. Tear ducts are activated in extreme circumstances causing continued oxygen intake struggle, resulting in a moist, red or purple face.

In his book, *Laughter: A Scientific Investigation*, world's leading scientific laughter expert, Dr. Robert R. Provine stated "Laughter is instinctive behavior programmed by our genes, not by the vocal community in which we grow up." Provine mentioned laughter disappears when he is ready to observe it -- especially in the lab. One study observed laughter's sonic structure. He discovered that human laughter consists of variations of short, vowel-like notes (syllables) repeated every 210 milliseconds. You may hear the notes "ha-ha-ha" or "ho-ho-ho" but not both. Provine suggests humans have a laugh "detector"- "a neural circuit in our brain that responds exclusively to laughter." When this is triggered, it generates more laughter, helping explain why laughter is contagious.

Dr. Provine suggests the following 10 tips to increase laughter: 1) Find a friend or personable stranger. 2) The more people to laugh with the merrier. 3) Increase interpersonal contact. 4) Create a casual atmosphere. 5) Adopt a laugh ready attitude. 6) Exploit the contagious laugh effect. 7) Provide humorous materials. 8) Remove social inhibitions. 9) Stage social events. 10) Tickle.

Osho also speaks about the power of laughter by stating "Laughter is a great medicine. It is a tremendously powerful therapy. If you can laugh at your own unconscious, the unconscious loses its force. In your very laughter, your guilt, your wounds, disappear."

LIFE

"Life is an aspiration. Its mission is to strive after perfection which is self-realization. The ideal must not be lowered because of our weaknesses or imperfections."
Mahatma Gandhi

Mahatma Gandhi said, "To believe in something and not to live it is dishonest." What do you aspire to be, do, have in life? How many believe in a better life yet live in a way, in a pool of habits that support the opposite? How many recognize they are not living from a place of integrity or greatness? How many are willing to reflect and do something about it?

As Oprah once stated "Life always whispers at first, if you ignore the whispers, life screams." Clues, messages, synchronicities are there to teach you, to inspire you and to tell you- move, do something different than what you were doing. What are you ignoring in your life and why? While it may appear easier to ignore things that are unpleasant or that you wish to not deal with, at some time, you must deal with them. You cannot run from yourself, no matter what country you escape to or how much work you do.

Invitation to expand:
Bob Proctor invited us to take a piece of white paper and realize this is our day. You begin each day with a blank canvas and it is up to you to paint it how you choose. What will you sculpt on that paper? How will you live your day? Euripides reminded you that wisdom comes from living life in balance. He stated "The best and safest thing is to keep a balance in your life, acknowledge the great powers around us and in us." Live in balance in your thoughts, feelings and actions.

WHAT IS LIFE?

"Life is an opportunity, benefit from it.
Life is a beauty, admire it.
Life is a dream, realize it.
Life is a challenge, meet it.
Life is a duty, complete it.
Life is a game, play it.
Life is a promise, fulfill it.
Life is sorrow, overcome it.
Life is a song, sing it.
Life is a struggle, accept it.
Life is a tragedy, confront it.
Life is an adventure, dare it.
Life is luck, make it.
Life is life, fight for it!"
- Mother Teresa

LISTEN/LISTENING

Rumi reminds you "Since in order to speak, one must first listen, learn to speak by listening."

Sound expert, Julian Treasure, during a July 2011 TEDGlobal talk in Edinburg, Scotland shared wonderful insight about listening. He stated that "We spend 60% of communication listening yet retain 25% of what we hear." He defines listening as "making meaning from sound."

Treasure shared the following 5 techniques of conscious listening:

1) "Silence" - 3 min a day of silence. 2) Mixer entails listening to how many individual sounds channels can hear. 3) "Savoring" involves enjoying mundane sounds like the clothes dryer. 4) "Listening positions" he states is the most important. This involves playing with the various filters (culture, language, etc.) and moving them to various positions. Examples include "active/passive, "reductive/expansive and critical/empathetic." 5) RASA, a Sanskrit word for juice, stands for Receive (pay attention), Appreciate (by making noises like hmm), Summarize and Ask many and good questions.

LOVE

"We must look deeply in order to see and understand the needs, aspirations and suffering of the person we love. This is the ground of real love. You cannot resist loving another person when you really understand him or her."
Thich Nhat Hanh

What is love? In Dr. Deepak Chopra's book, *The Path to Love*, he included a beautiful description of love:

> "Love is meant to heal.
> Love is meant to renew.
> Love is meant to make us safe.
> Love is meant to make us certain, without doubt.
> Love is meant to oust all fear.
> Love is meant to unveil immortality.
> Love is meant to bring peace.
> Love is meant to harmonize differences."

In *The Path to Love*, Dr. Chopra stated "To see love in the moment, you must close the windows of perception." He mentioned that when you know you are love, you will be in love. What are the ways you perceive love? Is it something you withhold, waiting for another to offer it first or do you give love freely, from your heart to yourself and everyone around you? When you feel love, speak truthfully from your heart and stay open. Dr. Chopra also stated "The awakening of true love lies in finding peace within passion and passion within peace."

June Masters Bacher stated "Love is like a violin. The music may stop now and then but the strings remain forever." Understanding you are love and full of love is vital to life. This awareness is profound and moves you from a place of desperation to a place of inspiration. Dr. Chopra reminds you, "Three things are absolute and cannot be destroyed: awareness, being and love."

"If you look at the great religions, they may not agree on karma and afterlife and this and that but all of them agree on one thing, when you strip it down to the core. That one thing is essential-Love. It's the very core of what you and I are." Kute Blackson, speaker, life coach.

Dr. Richard Gerber, author of *Vibrational Medicine* discovered the most powerful healing force in the universe is unconditional love. In an interview with Edward Brown, he stated when you work from that level, you increase discovery of self-exploration and spiritual transformation. You begin a new level of healing, fixing the body and moving to a new understanding of your life and awareness as an evolving spiritual being.

Invitation to expand:

As Kute Blackson says: "It's time for us all to step up and love now. I invite you to this challenge; I invite you to this new possibility of loving NOW." Surround yourself with love and loving people. Be loving and you will attract more love into your life.

"ME FILE"

Recently, I read about a concept, introduced by Michael Josephson of www.charactercounts.org, called a "Me" File. Sally Kinnamon shared this concept with him. She suggested you label a folder "Me File" and place in it all complimentary cards, notes, letters and performance reviews. Whenever you feel unappreciated or undervalued, open this file and read the correspondence.

MEDITATION

"Meditation is the foundation of neural reconditioning process and the ground upon which you build structures of new beliefs, goals and aspirations in your nonconscious mind."
John Assaraf and Murray Smith, in the book *The Answers*

What is meditation? Osho stated "Meditation is a state of total relaxation; not of concentration, not of contemplation, but of relaxation.

When one is so absolutely relaxed that there is no tension in the body or in the mind, suddenly there is an opening of the heart." Meditation allows you to expand your awareness, your consciousness and go beyond your current physical paradigms. It allows you to quiet your mind. According to John Assaraf and Murray Smith, meditation helps build new beliefs, goals and aspirations in the subconscious mind. Dr. Kabat-Zin reminds you that the practice of non-doing or meditating is vital as the world becomes more complicated. Joan Borysenko, Ph.D. stated "Meditation helps to keep us from identifying with the movies of the mind."

In addition to quieting your mind and expanding your awareness, meditation offers many health benefits. Dr. Deepak Chopra stated, "Numerous studies show the many health benefits of meditation including lowered blood pressure, stress reduction and increased immune function."

The following are types of meditation and may help you relax and focus. The two general types of meditation that exist are concentrative and mindfulness meditation. Concentrative meditation focuses attention on breath, an image or sound (mantra), to still the mind and allow greater awareness. Sitting quietly, focusing attention on breath is the simplest form of concentrative meditation. Many who practice yoga and meditation believe a correlation exists between breath and mind state. For example, an anxious, frightened and agitated person tends to breathe rapidly, uneven and shallow. However, a person with a clear, calm and focused mind tends to have slow, deep and regular breaths. As you focus your awareness on breath, your mind is absorbed in the rhythm of inhalation and exhalation.

According to Dr. Borysenko, mindfulness meditation "Involves opening the attention to become aware of the continuously passing parade of sensations and feelings, images, thoughts, sounds, smells and so forth without becoming involved in thinking about them." Sit quietly and witness whatever occupies the mind without reacting or involving thoughts, memories, worries or images. This helps clear the mind, allowing for an awareness of the Universe.

One example of meditation includes Vipassana Meditation, an ancient Indian technique. According to www.dharma.org, Vipassana means to see things as they really are. More than 2500 years ago, Gotama Buddha rediscovered it and taught it as a remedy for universal ills. Through Vipassana, one's self-observation leads to self-transformation. Life is characterized by increased awareness, non-delusion, self-control and peace of mind. Through 10 days of complete silence; meditation and observation of mind-body; how suffering is produced and released is understood.

MIND/BODY INTERACTION

"The mind is like a sponge. We squeeze it hard with our anxious thoughts but not until we can release the pressure and allow the sponge to take its normal shape can it become absorbent and receptive again."
Dr. Raymond Holliwell

What is your mind full of? Mike Dooley, author of *Infinite Possibilities,* stated "If you want love, happiness, health or wealth, create it first in your mind." Sue and Aaron Singleton, founders of The Way To Balance, developed Energy of Life (EOL) Process to promote the healing of "physical, emotional and spiritual manifestations of dis-ease." I was fortunate to engage in this training and grew tremendously. Some highlights include: enhancing intuition; understanding self-diagnosis; root cause determination and activating this process in others. I highly recommend EOL to all interested in a life changing view of the mind/body connection.

Bob Proctor echoes Allen's words with "Body is an instrument of my mind. Mind is movement. Body is the manifestation of that movement." When you review these words, it is evident that what you think affects your body. Your thoughts tell the body how to respond, whether you choose these thoughts consciously or not, the body obeys.

Louise L. Hay, in her book *Heal Your Body,* explains how negative thoughts become diseases in the body. Some examples include: "constipation arises from refusing to let go of old ideas; coughs arise from irritating thoughts not spoken and deafness occurs from a desire not to listen." In addition, your physical environment may contribute to disease. If you feed your body, healthy nourishing food and thoughts, you encourage the maintenance of a healthy body. Candace Pert, in her book, *Molecules of Emotion* refers to Elmer Green's quote below (which summarizes the above well). Green stated,

SOUL INGREDIENTS

"Every change in the physiological state is accompanied by an appropriate change in the mental-emotional state, conscious or unconscious, and every change in the mental-emotional state is accompanied by an appropriate change in the physiological state."

Osho reiterates this stating the body affects the mind and the mind affects the body. He expressed, "You are not body "and" mind, you are bodymind, psychosomatic." You are both mind and body simultaneously. When you suppress something in your mind, your body suppresses it (which, after many years, may lead to your entire body becoming diseased). In Chinese medicine, it is understood that chi that does not flow may lead to blood problems and further complications. However, if your mind releases everything, your body will also release everything.

MISTAKES

"Every mistake we made occurred because in moment we made it, we were not in conscious contact with our highest self. We were not centered in spirit. This is why making contact and spending time daily fostering it is the most powerful thing we can do."
Marianne Williamson, from *Gift of Change: Spiritual Guidance for Living Your Best Life*

Bob Proctor mentioned "Every time you lose or make a mistake, it's an education." Mistakes are best approached with humor and insight. Recognize that all mistakes, as Proctor stated, are learning lessons. This thought is reiterated by Rev. Michael B. Beckwith. In his book *Spiritual Liberation,* Beckwith reflects on mistakes stating, "Your willingness to take the risk of making a mistake is actually an expression of courage and a willingness to grow from them. Mistakes are about getting the blessing in the lesson and the lesson in the blessing."

MOTIVATION

"Trust is the highest form of human motivation."
Stephen R. Covey

You can perform the right actions with the wrong motivation. Be careful of this for you may recognize the virtue in doing the right things yet may be blinded with a motivation that is not in integrity. The motivation affects the action.

Invitation to expand:
In the *Edgar Cayce Ideals Workbook* by Kevin Todeschi, Todeschi mentioned noticing motivations for decision making. For 30 days, Todeschi suggests making a list of daily experiences and what motivated you to make them. List the decision on the left side of the page and the motivation for decision making on the right. An example includes not cleaning the house. A motivation for this decision may be laziness. At the end of 30 days, notice what happened. What differences do you see in your thinking and experiences?

MOVEMENT

"The most important factor for survival, after water, air, salt and food is exercise."
F. Batmanghelidg, MD

Edward Stanley reminds you, "Those who think they have no time for bodily exercise will sooner or later have to find time for illness." Many types of physical movement can be enjoyed from walking, running, cycling, hiking, pilates, swimming and yoga. Whatever activity you partake in, make it fun and enjoy it. Not only will you feel better, you will be motivated to take part in it again.

A suggestion to incorporate movement into a busy life includes combining it with other elements of life. For example, as a parent, you place your kids in a stroller and push the stroller while running. Finding ways to combine family time with physical movement is brilliant and brings the family closer in spirit and health. It also teaches kids healthy habits and moves energy, blood and cells as nature intended.

MUSIC

"The new sound-sphere is global. It ripples at great speed across languages, ideologies, frontiers and races. The economics of this musical Esperanto is staggering. Rock and pop breed concentric worlds of fashion, setting and life-style. Popular music has brought with it sociologies of private and public manner, of group solidarity. The politics of Eden come loud."
George Steiner

Deanna Phelps and Stephen Hager, co-founders of The Hadron Group, brain based human development products and founders of Brain PathWays™… The Neuroscience of You (the most advanced practical neuroscience product for daily living), state that MUSIC can accelerate creativity, learning and memory. Singer, songwriter and LMT Karyn Grant stated "Music is a form of ''light' and has healing vibrations of its own."

Below are two eloquently written pieces about music. The first comes from Olivea Dewhurst-Maddock's book entitled *The Book of Sound Therapy* and the second from musician and composer Robert Haig Coxon who began playing piano with both hands at 1 ½ years old.

The Book of Sound Therapy by Olivea Dewhurst-Maddock states "The human being is therefore likened to a very complex and finely tuned musical instrument. Every atom, molecule, cell, tissue and organ of the body continually broadcasts the frequencies of physical, emotional, mental and spiritual life. The human voice is an indicator of its body's health on all these levels of existence. It establishes a relationship between the individual and the wondrous network of vibrations that is the cosmos."

Robert Haig Coxon, in a blog on his website www.robertcoxon.com stated: "Madame Blavetski and Rudolf Steiner hold that uplifting music comes from a spiritual source and that its vibrations have an uplifting effect that puts us in touch with our true essence. Gurdjieff, as the ancient Greeks Aristotle and Plato did, related music to the cosmos, connecting us with Universal order and Universal consciousness. In all great civilizations music was of ultimate importance, deriving its energy from above for the working of change below. The role of Sacred Music was to release on earth a form of energy that could keep civilization in harmony with the heavens."

Music is sacred and transforms one to another time and place. Each type of music vibrates at a unique frequency and affects all it encounters differently. Think of how you feel listening to classical music. Is it relaxing? For some it invokes a sleep state. Now imagine a different musical scene- a heavy metal concert. It is a much different experience than classical with a different frequency. How does heavy metal music make you feel?

The following, taken from an article entitled, *The Secret Connections Between Music and Performance Excellence* from the blog http://blog.brainpathways.net/tag/classical-music, are suggestions you may wish to incorporate into your life:

For Active Learning- read aloud or silently to the beat of the music.

Mozart (According to Don Campbell, Mozart strengthens the mind.)

Brahms: Violin Concerto in D major

Beethoven: Concerto #5 for piano – E Flat major, Concerto for Violin in D major

For Memorizing- play this music while reading (aloud or silently) material to memorize for meetings, negotiations, presentations, trainings or exams.

Bach: Brandenburg Concertos, Preludes and Fugues for Organ

Vivaldi: The Four Seasons, Five Concertos for Flute

Handel: Water Music, Royal Fireworks Music

To enhance Creativity - play the following while solving problems, "brainstorming," writing, engaging in artwork or inventing.

Tchaikovsky, P.: The Nutcracker Suite

Claude Debussy: La mer, Prelude a l'apres midi d'un Faun

Ravel: Daphne et Chloe

Other suggestions are listening to and singing songs with empowering words like Daybreak Song, written by Jewel's mom, Lenedra J. Carroll. When I sang this song with Lenedra and 300 others, it resonated with me that I, like her, sing it daily. For more information, view www.lenedracarroll.com.

Daybreak Song begins with:

"I will give this breath to the rising sun,
to the day that follows and the night to come.
May I work with Spirit, knowing all are one
and I will that thy will be done."

Invitation to expand:
As beings, whether you are professionally trained and call yourself a musician or not, you create music daily. There is music in the way you live your life, the way you walk, the way you talk. What music are you creating today? Is it uplifting?

NATURE

Guy Finley, in his Seven Steps to Oneness audio, spoke about why humans like nature so much. He stated "When you experience the air, a beautiful bird, in those moments, what makes it breathtaking is the usual mind's story is suspended because when you see clouds, sunrise, something so true and pure, in that same moment, what I have seen, for stillness or belief in it, that exterior quality resonates and stirs interior in me, its story. In that moment I am not in a story of my own. My mind becomes quiet in great moments of beauty."

NOW

"Present moment is made up of the past and is substance of which the future will be made. Past is there in the form of the present. If touch the present deeply, can heal the past."
Thich Nhat Hanh

Time is an illusion of the linear mind and the attachment to it does not allow you to be free. Only the Now exists. In Eckhart Tolle's book, *The Power of Now*, he stated "The more you are focused on time-past and present, the more you miss the Now, the most precious thing there is."
This may be difficult for some to grasp. Tolle clarified it asking "Have you ever experienced, done, thought or felt anything outside the Now?"

The answer is no. The future is what you imagine it and the past is a former Now. Therefore, what is here is the Now. When you stop ruminating in the past and stop trying to grasp the future, you enjoy this moment, the Now. You become ever present to its magnificence and all possibilities. Colors appear brighter and the essence of nature, music and people magnifies.

How do you access the power of Now? I invite you to practice withdrawing attention from the past and the future. Observe, without judgment, your mind, thoughts and emotions as they wander to the past and to the future. Realize that you are not present and in this awareness, you become present to the Now. Tolle also suggested yielding to life's flow or accepting the moment as it is Now and not going against it. He reminds you that "Guilt, regret, resentment, sadness, bitterness and nonforgiveness are all caused by too much past and not enough presence. You cannot be both unhappy and fully present in the Now."

Sharon Stone, in the book *Ten Eternal Questions* gave this advice when author Zoë Sallis asked her about wisdom "Remember that your whole life is just this minute. This is your life, live widely and fully and plenteously, in the now."

ONENESS

"Whatever affects one directly,
Affects all indirectly...
This is the interrelated structure of reality."
Martin Luther King Jr.

In Guy Finley's audio recording, *Seven Steps to Oneness: Journey to a Whole New Life*, he spoke about oneness. He stated "Oneness is a never ending story. Your true nature is created in this force of love whether you see it or not. We need to bring ourselves back to the present moment where this presence lives and for whose presence in us we are given a glimpse of all it created with us to work on and change, it begins to do things we've been unable to do." Have you ever experienced a sense of oneness with something, whether it was nature, a scientific concept or a person? In that moment of oneness, nothing limits you, the Universe is wide open. No fears cloud your vision, no pressure is upon you. You flow, effortless, like a river. Your connection to the infinite is within you and you are connected to everything in this quantum universe. Rev. Michael B. Beckwith reminds you "Everything affects everything."

Ramana Maharshi, a great Indian spiritual master, once said "God, Guru and Self are ultimately One." This One lies beyond the many and encompasses all. It is infinite and all knowing.

In *Book III, Conversations with God*, Neale Donald Walsch stated "To remain in the state of sublime no-thing, or Oneness with the All, would make it impossible to be there. As I've just explained, That Which Is cannot be, except in the space of That Which is Not. The total bliss of Oneness cannot be experienced as "total bliss" unless something less than total bliss exists. Something less than total bliss of total Oneness had to be- and continually has to be-created."

OPPORTUNITIES

"The greatest achievement of the human spirit is to live up to one's opportunities and make the most of one's resources."
Luc De Clapiers

Dave Weinbaum stated "A window of opportunity won't open itself." In other words, you must recognize opportunity and act upon it. Some suggest creating your own opportunities. Sun Tzu suggested "Opportunities multiply as they are seized." As you partake in more and more opportunities, you build momentum and attract their energy and ways to serve others. Coming from a place of recognition allows you to create more opportunities. In a creative state, anything is possible.

PAIN

"Everybody feels pain and everybody feels it for a different reason on a different day in a different way. It's all real....there's no pain that isn't valid, there's no pain that isn't "real" because

somebody has it worse off. All you can do is feel it, accept it, move on and know everybody else on this spinning ball of dirt is in the same boat. We all need to acknowledge each other's pain; no matter what the package and no matter how big or small that package appears. When we do this, that's what keeps us compassionate brothers and sisters on earth. "

Amanda F. Palmer of *Grand Theft Orchestra*, blog post

Dr. James Tin Yau So, ND, Lic. Ac and founder of New England School of Acupuncture (NESA) stated "Pain is afraid of me- when it sees me coming it runs the other way." Is pain afraid of you or does it run toward you whenever you experience heartache, disappointment or anything you deem negative? As Kenji Miyazawa stated "We must embrace pain and burn it as fuel for our journey." Only then, may you move through your pain into a space of acceptance and gratitude.

Invitation to expand:
Pain is part of life and some believe, as Victor Campbell told me in 2008 that "We learn how to be a leader through our pain." While this may be true, it is important to tune into another frequency, of non- judgment, love and acceptance to alleviate pain and as Amanda Palmer stated, "Acknowledge each person's pain."

In *Conversations With God, Book I*, Neale Donald Walsch stated "Nothing is painful in and of itself. Pain is the result of wrong thought. It is an error in thinking. Pain results from a judgment you made about a thing. Remove that judgment and the pain disappears." There is no reason to live in pain and there is no reason to make excuses because of pain. Live life fully, in the present moment, in bliss, gratitude and inspiration. Let the pain of the physical, emotional and spirit bodies be a passing thought on your daily voyage of love.

PARADIGMS

"Your paradigms create the magnetic field."
Mary Morrissey

SOUL INGREDIENTS

In *The 7 Habits of Highly Effective People,* Stephen Covey described a paradigm as "A model, a theory, perception, assumption or frame of reference. It is the way we "see" the world, in terms of our perceiving, understanding and interpreting."

Bob Proctor reintroduced paradigms to me in 2009. He stated "You must have a goal more powerful than your paradigm." In other words, paradigms are fixed ideas or beliefs or a way of conditioning that live in the subconscious. Paradigms are formed by: thoughts, images and ideas that come from parents, caregivers, friends, society and may not be evident. Fixed ideas become paradigms, becoming fixed beliefs and habits.

Napoleon Hill stated it well with, "Our only limitations are those we set up in our minds." An example is someone who grew up in a home and was told there is not enough food, money, etc. As the person grows up, he/she may have a 'lack' mentality. Lack mentality repeats so that person says he/she doesn't have enough $$ to go out, etc. This translates to daily actions, decisions, etc. based on these fixed ideas.

Another way to view paradigms is the concept of a broken record, continuously playing, regardless of what transpires. For example, you may read and the thought "I am too old. I am not smart enough" circulates throughout your mind.

How do you change paradigms? It is important to first understand they exist and secondly, form a positive attitude toward them. As mentioned earlier, attitude is a combination of thoughts, feelings and actions. A powerful action step to change paradigms is to daily replace them with life affirming ideas. (See Affirmations) Suggestions include: examining why you feel the way you do and understanding who influenced you. Is that your thought or that of your parents, sisters, husband, wife, etc.? Also, you may choose to not think about it and clear it energetically. Your choice is unique and depends on where your path is and what resonates with you.

To change these ideas took time and a willingness to understand the how and why of it. Once I acknowledged this and that everyone in my life did their best with what they knew at the space and time they were in (and their paradigms), the energy toward my paradigms shifted. Judgment was gone and in its place flowed unconditional love (spanning years of inner work and one of my most rewarding challenges). As Iyanla Vanzant stated, "Once

I forgive me, there is no one else to forgive". Daily, I repeat affirmations to replace prior ideas that do not serve me. Also, I often recognize the pattern before it plays out.

Often, when clients of www.pagona.com embrace their true selves and let go of preconceived notions, their fixed 'understanding' changes as well as their consistent action, firm beliefs and application of truth. This manifests in those around them being 'different', often with no understanding of what transpired. (See Universal Laws).

You are capable of ALL you think (even if you do not think you are). Step outside your fears, preconditioned beliefs and anything that does not serve you and your highest good and OWN your true power. Once you step inside this empowered reality, life becomes magical...

PASSION/PURPOSE

"Every problem in life is a question trying to ask itself. Every question in life is an answer trying to reveal itself. Every action in life is a way of life trying to be born."
Rev. Michael B. Beckwith in *The Answer is You*

James Allen stated "Until thought is linked with purpose, there is no intelligent accomplishment." You have a purpose in life that you may question. What and who will you serve? What kind of person will you be? For me, passion is a precursor to purpose as it is important to do what you are passionate about to serve your true, authentic purpose. You may work in areas you are passionate about yet find something is missing. Passion and a deep inner knowing both serve your purpose. How do you find your passion or purpose?

Invitation to expand:
Oprah Winfrey reminds you, "Your true passion should feel like breathing; it's that natural." What do you love to do? What do you do that while doing it time passes without staring at the clock? What legacy do you wish to leave for your children and humanity? Who and what will you build your life around? You may wish to seek out and find your true calling, your purpose, your passion and live life according to that. It is then that your life

will reflect a true alignment with the Divine.

PATIENCE

"Patience is no small, feel-good personal quality. It is at the heart of diplomacy and civility, lawfulness and civil order. Without it, people can't work together and society can't function at all. With it, we create the possibility of peace between people and between nations."
Mary Jane Ryan, *The Power of Patience*

My first and true understanding of patience occurred in Spain. I was backpacking throughout Europe alone and finally arrived at a hostel in Spain. The pleasant woman behind the desk looked at the anxious, tired crowd of young people in front of her and asked "Do you have patience?" I was quick to respond with "Yes" to which she uttered "Use it." This remained with me throughout the years as I 'use' patience daily. It is a story often retold to illustrate a simple yet profound choice.

Patience is a virtue and choice. It is something you choose to embrace and quiet your mind or choose not to yield to and thus engage in life's chaos.

PEACEFUL CONFLICT RESOLUTION

"Peace is not something you wish for; it's something you make, something you do, something you are, something you give away."
Robert Fulghum, Author

In the documentary, *Prey the Devil Back to Hell,* the women of Liberia ended a 10 year civil war by peaceful protest and non-cooperation. Daily, 3,000 women gathered, pressing Charles Taylor, Liberia's leader at that time and his rebels to end violence. Bringing together women of different faiths and tribes, 'no' was not an option for them. They succeeded after Leymah Gibowee, about to be arrested, told 'security': "I'm going to strip naked." In West Africa, to see a woman publically strip naked is believed to be a curse.

Two weeks later, a peace treaty was announced.

Ellen Johnson Sirleaf became Africa's first elected head of state in 2006 as Liberia's president. Although Liberia has widespread poverty and many areas have poor infrastructure with no running water and electricity, the situation is improving.

By peacefully resolving this conflict, the 3,000 women in Liberia inhabit a different land called home. This is one example of many of how peaceful conflict resolution resolves issues without violence. John Lennon, sang it well in this excerpt from the song Revolution:

"You say you want a revolution
Well now you know
We all want to change the world
You tell me that it's evolution
But when you talk about destruction
Don't you know that you can count me out
You better free you mind instead."

According to www.sgi.org, Soka Gakkai or Nichiren Buddhism is another way to promote peace. Soka Gakkai International (SGI) has a global network of independent SGI organizations in 90 countries and territories. SGI teaches the philosophy and practice of Nichiren Buddhism which promotes "the causes of peace, culture and education in their respective societies, while the organization also developed large-scale international public exhibitions on such issues as building a culture of peace, nuclear abolition, sustainable development and human rights." This Buddhist philosophy focuses on transformation of the individual instead of solely societal reforms.

Daisaku Ikeda, president of Soka Gakkai wrote a book entitled, *The Human Revolution* in which he described Soka Gakkai's history and ideals. A quote from that book reads: "A great inner revolution in just a single individual will help achieve a change in the destiny of a nation and further, enable a change in the destiny of all humankind."

In *Book II of Conversations With God,* Neale Donald Walsh mentions that "Love breeds tolerance, tolerance breeds peace. The fastest way to get to a place of love and concern for all humankind is to see all humankind as your family." A solution is offered in lieu of war which entails every human on the planet seeking and finding internal peace. In this way, Walsch states to strive to see the perfection in everything; need nothing and desire everything and "In the middle of the greatest tragedy, see the glory in the process." This is the change of consciousness needed.

For those who believe nothing can be done in the world today, perhaps your awareness of the above helps you see something once unseen. You are witnessing an increase in global awareness regarding peaceful conflict resolutions that do not include loss of humanity. Perhaps you forgot how important, you, combined with many of 'you' are in the global village we call humanity.

Mahatma Gandhi and Martin Luther King Jr. opposed injustice, irrationality and war with a firm confrontation full of love and compassion that embraced everyone. You have much to learn from them and leaders following their footsteps. Martin Luther King Jr. once said "Love is the only force capable of transforming an enemy into a friend."

PERCEPTION

"Rather than demand from each person qualities he doesn't possess…What if we choose, instead, to NURTURE those positive traits he does have? Not only does our perception change but so does our world."
Sue and Aaron Singleton, founders of
www.thewaytobalance.com

A physics principle called Heisenberg states "When you change the way you look at something, the thing you look at changes in response." Like Sue and Aaron's quote above, your world changes when your perception changes. With an open mind, all things are possible. All things may be understood as willingness exists to know and comprehend. Nothing is blocked from your view. Truth is allowed in. Henri Bergson tells you, "The eyes see only what the mind is prepared to comprehend." Allow the mind to understand, keep it open like a parachute and truly see. What do you notice that is different?

When you see yourself, in your mind's eye healthy and full of energy, you become healthy and feed your body and soul nutritious food. Your perception or paradigm is one embodying health instead of sickness. Perceive the image you desire in your mind and watch it unfold.

PERSISTENCE (PLEASANTLY PERSISTENT)

"You have to develop mental strength. You develop mental strength with the will. The will is the mental faculty that gives you the ability to hold one idea under the screen of your mind to the exclusion of all outside distractions."
Bob Proctor

Emerson stated "That which we persist in doing becomes easier, not that the nature of the task changed but our ability to do has increased." By daily exercising your will; persistence and focused attention, life becomes more enjoyable. Your concentration increases and things are accomplished with greater ease. Remember to be pleasantly persistent.

PINEAL GLAND

The Source Field Investigations: The Hidden Science and Lost Civilizations Behind the 2012 Prophecies by David Wilcock, states, "Many different ancient traditions say there is a physical gland deep within the center of the brain, where telepathic thought transmissions and visual images are received." The pineal gland is believed to be the first point of contact for telepathic information exchange. It has been called the seat of the soul. For Hindus, the pineal is the Third Eye; for Buddhists it is the all- seeing eye and Christianity refers to it as the eye single.

According to information in *The Source Field Investigations*, the pineal gland accumulates fluoride (has the highest concentration in the body) and produces serotonin. A study in the Journal of Pineal Research revealed "Many problems could be caused by pineal calcification and malfunction including depression, anxiety, eating disorders and mental illness."

POSSIBILITIES

"Remember you can do anything, big or small, facile or difficile that you, a human capable of many great feats, allow, set, free and discipline your mind to do."
Pagona while I studied for an Organic Chemistry exam in college.

Raymond Holliwell states "Always make it a point of moving forward in your mind, ever seeking to unfold your power of thought and to develop hidden possibilities." When you continue to think, to harness ideas and the power of the mind in a positive way, you are full of possibilities. The world is open. Possibilities exist everywhere for those who resonate at that frequency. Think of what you can do instead of what cannot be done. If you think it is not possible, it will not be. Conversely, if you think it is possible, it will be.

PRACTICE

"That which transforms your life is what you practice. What you practice, you ultimately embody, paving the way for breakthroughs; insights; fresh realizations and evolutions of consciousness."
Taken from the film *Spiritual Liberation*

Martha Graham shared a wonderful definition and example of practice with, "I believe that we learn by practice. Whether it means to learn to dance by practicing dancing or to learn to live by practicing living, the principles are the same. In each, it is the performance of a dedicated precise set of acts, physical or intellectual, from which comes shape of achievement, a sense of one's being, a satisfaction of spirit. Practice means to perform, over and over again in the face of all obstacles, some act of vision, of faith, of desire. Practice is a means of inviting the perfection desired." I invite you to make a daily effort to use what you learn to make progress and realize your dreams. Practice, therefore, is a fundamental component of all endeavors.

Invitation to expand:

During his 29 July 2012 service at Agape Spiritual Center, Rev. Michael B. Beckwith stated "Practice triumphs belief." What practices do you partake in daily? What do you make yourself available to? How can you ensure your practice is greater than your negative beliefs?

PRAYER

"Water carries within it your thoughts and prayers. As you yourself are water, no matter where you are your prayers will be carried to the rest of the world."
Masaru Emoto in *The Secret Life of Water*

Dr. Raymond Holliwell shared, "Praise is the shortest route to complete any demonstration and the quickest way to enjoy effectual prayer." If you review the Law of Attraction, you understand that like Holliwell stated, you attract what you think or what you create. Speaking and living in a vibration of praise creates more praise. This frequency attracts more things to be thankful for. You create an environment of goodness and spark the abundance in the Universe.

According to an article by Alice Dembner, for thousands of years, people of various faiths used and continue to use prayer for the sick. She states that in America, prayer is the most frequently used form of alternative medicine.

Although scientists attempt to study the effects of prayer on patient health, it is not easily quantifiable. Often prayer and other forms of energy healing are misunderstood as many are unaware that energy exists everywhere simultaneously. Dr. Mitchell Krucoff, professor of medicine and cardiology at Duke University stated that [prayer] "Is the most ancient, widely practiced therapy on the face of the earth." Dr. Krucoff mentioned that various faiths including Catholic, Judaism and Muslim include prayers for the sick as part of their regular services.

Susan Misselbeck is sure prayer helped her daughter Courtney Ridd when she underwent a liver transplant after battling a rare liver disease. Misselbeck said her Jewish friends said prayers in synagogues. People of different faiths across the country - many unknown to Misselbeck, prayed for her daughter. Courtney, now 28, is well. Misselbeck stated "That powerful energy gave us a sense of peace. It felt like a nice warm blanket, wrapping us in it, saying it's going to be O.K."

Ascended Master Saint Germain stated "Pray as if everything depends on us and act as if everything depends on you." The 'us' he refers to is angels, guides and loved ones. Whether you believe in them is not important. Understanding prayer can have a profound impact is important. Experiment with it and see for yourself.

PROGRESS

"There must be a constant stream of new thought, better thought and truer thought to insure progression in life."
Dr. Raymond Holliwell

Stephen Covey, in *The 7 Habits of Highly Effective People,* stated "To keep progressing, we must learn, commit and do-learn, commit and do again." If you learn yet do not apply, much progress cannot be made. Likewise if you learn and apply and fail to learn more, this will hinder true progress. Daily thinking, questioning, learning and applying are important.

QUESTION

"He who asks is a fool for 5 minutes but he who does not ask remains a fool forever."
Chinese proverb

I am often heard saying "If you don't ask the question, the answer is always no." If you ask, you have a chance of yes. How will you know, if the question is not posed. Remember the quality of your questions determines the quality of your answers.

Deepak Chopra, MD, at an IIN conference in 2011, shared 10 questions with the audience. He suggested reflecting daily upon one of the following:

PAGONA

1. **"Who am I?**
2. What do I want?
3. What is a peak experience for me?
4. What's my life purpose?
5. What kind of contribution do I want to make to society and the world?
6. What does a meaningful relationship look like to me?
7. How do I contribute to relationships I have?
8. What are my unique skills and talents and how do I use them to serve humanity?
9. Who are my heroines and heroes in history, mythology and religion?
10. What is my story?"

RACE

"The smallest minority on earth is the individual. Those who deny individual rights cannot claim to be defenders of minorities."
Ayn Rand

Nigerian writer, Chimamanda Ngozi Adichie wrote "The single story creates stereotypes and the problem with stereotypes is not that they are untrue, but that they are incomplete. They make one story become the only story." Once the world is explained based on his/her story and excludes the possibility of other's stories, separation occurs and therefore, understanding cannot occur.

James Earl Jones stated "Once you begin to explain or excuse all events on racial grounds, you begin to indulge in the perilous mythology of race." A large component of traveling, for me, continues to be about listening to and embracing global stories from anyone and everyone. When I choose to be present and listen to what I hear, see and feel, the concept of race as we know it ceases to exist.

Invitation to expand:
During my travels, I developed a habit I continue today. When meeting

people, I automatically wonder what country they hail from. In my mind, as I'm talking with them, I guess the country and when I say it out loud, most of the time it is correct. Why would I do this? It forms a connection and bond that helps people become comfortable and open. It is done with enthusiasm as I understand we are all one. This one habit continues to help me in all aspect of life, both professionally and socially.

If this does not resonate with you, find a similar habit that helps you connect with others that 'appear' unlike you. You may attempt to speak their language or embrace their food. Whatever you choose, do it with love and compassion as your intent will shine. When humanity embraces similarities within a space of love and compassion, unloving acts diminish and a world of harmony re-emerges. Nigerian writer, Chinua Achebe, wrote "As long as one people sit on another and are deaf to their cry, so long will understanding and peace elude all of us." Be open and understanding and receptive to others for they are your mirrors.

READING

"No matter how busy you may think you are, you must find time for reading, or surrender yourself to self-chosen ignorance."
Confucius

Edmund Burk once said "Reading without reflecting is like eating without digesting." How many read because you must for school, work or otherwise? In the process, do you read as fast as possible to finish the assignment to do something else? What if you read because you desire to learn and grow your mind? What if you incorporated it as a daily habit, having fun while reflecting upon the words read? I like to say "Reading is like dreaming, both transport you to the inner recesses of your mind."

Lyndon Baines Johnson stated "A book is the most effective weapon against intolerance and ignorance." Anna Quindlen shared, "Books are the plane, the train and the road. They are the destination and the journey, They are home."

Invitation to expand:
Turn off the TV for 1 week and read a book. Reflect on what you

learned, understand and apply it. Share it with your wife, husband, girlfriend, boyfriend or friend. Alternatively, have a book night instead of date night and discuss key principles learned, implementing one principle weekly. For example, in *The 7 Habits of Highly Effective People,* Steven Covey discussed 7 Habits- one is seek first to understand then be understood. Understand your spouse, kids or friends before desiring they understand you.

RELATIONSHIPS

"Other people must be in alignment with our thoughts for there to be partnership, friendship or adversarial relationship. We can always find what we are looking for as long as we don't insist upon who it is. Imagine how you want to feel or end result of whatever it is you really want."
Mike Dooley author of *Infinite Possibilities*

Dr. Shaunti Feldhahn, in her book and survey *For Women Only,* asked "What is the most important thing you wish your wife/significant other knew but feel you can't explain it to her/him or tell her/him?" Quickly ponder that question and ask yourself why you haven't said it. Take action now. Tomorrow is not guaranteed since time is now. Do it now.

Michael Levine shared "Before you focus on finding the right person, concentrate on being the right person." If you would like to attract a loving, honest person, be loving and honest. If you would like to attract your beloved, be the beloved. Also, embracing the inherent difference of females and males helps you understand relationship better. In *Emotional Wellness,* Osho reminds you "The way of the heart is beautiful but dangerous; The way of the mind is ordinary but safe. The man chose the safest and most shortcut way of life. The woman chose the most beautiful but the most mountainous, dangerous path of emotions, sentiments and moods."

RESPONSIBILITY

You are all responsible for yourselves and the thoughts and actions you have. You are also responsible for the environment you create while interacting with others. Responsibility involves a commitment to self and an understanding that your reality is a mirror of your inner world.

For parents, you share a deeper responsibility to breathe your wisdom and knowledge into precious and wise little beings. It involves a melding of simultaneous surrender, acceptance, love and gratitude. There is nothing more precious than love with a healthy, joyous and peaceful soul.

Invitation to expand:

When and what did you decide to not take responsibility for? Is it your health, relationships, growth? How are you manifesting lack of responsibility in your daily journey?

Within your beautiful soul is housed infinite power that you have access to daily. You need only ask for the answers. YOU create your thoughts and all that comes to you. Your parents raised you with the knowledge they had, in the best manner they knew.

It is time to stop blaming, playing the victim and start owning-owning your thoughts, actions and power. No one is responsible for you except YOU. Use the tools in this book to get started.

Put down the blame and anger and embrace the wisdom and power of a life molded to your brilliant and empowering specifications. YOU ARE THE ARCHITECT OF YOUR LIFE. WHAT WILL YOU BUILD? Will you build rigid walls or castles of love? Will you embrace yourself and the beauty called you? Until you take responsibility for EVERYTHING you created, true healing may elude you.

SACRED KNOWLEDGE

"A path becomes a path by people walking it.
A thing being called something becomes it.
Why is it so?
It is because it is so.

PAGONA

Why is it not something other than what it is?
It is because it is not."

Zhuang Zi

Sacred knowledge of various cultures has a lot to offer. Many ancient civilizations including the Mayans were in tune with nature and life's biological cycles. Also, many, including the Chinese, practice ancestor worship, honoring the lives of those who passed on. In his book *The Great Ancestral Teacher*, Zhuang Zi stated, "There are those who know heaven and know humanity. Those who know heaven know that heaven gives one life. Whoever knows humanity uses knowing to nurture what cannot be known. They run out the string of their years and do not find it cut off in the middle. This is the fullest knowledge. Though this is so, there is a problem. Knowledge waits on certainty but certainty is never quite certain."

Yamomotos stated:
"What is to be reduced is 1st expanded,
What is to be weakened is 1st strengthened,
What is to be abolished is 1st established."

SELF

"I am playing with my Self, I am playing with the world's soul, and I am the dialogue between my Self and el espiritu del mundo. I change myself, I change the world."
Gloria Anzaldua, Tejana Chicana poet

A friend once shared something she heard yet didn't know the source. As soon as she said "What other people think of me is none of my business," I grasped its importance. Years later I understood the deeper layers of this statement and incorporated it into daily life. It is not that you don't care about them, it is how you feel about you that matters. When you do not care what others think of you, you focus on what YOU think of YOU.

In his book, *Descartes' Error*, neurologist Antonio Damasio, stated that a sense of self depends on integrating thinking and feeling and if this integration does not exist, it compromises decision making ability. Indecision often results from a difficulty connecting the two- feelings and thinking. Balanced emotions are critical for a healthy sense of self and everything in life.

Also, your beliefs are shaped by who you surround yourself with. Be mindful of this and know each soul is on his/her journey. As José Ortega y Gasset stated "The will to be oneself is heroism." Be yourself, listen to positive people and stay away from those who bring you down, in word, deed or action. On your journey being yourself, remember the words of Gamaliel Bailey "The first and worst of all frauds is to cheat oneself." Honor self and stay true to you, to the inner knowing, to the intuition that is screaming to be heard or whispering for attention.

Thich Nhat Hanh reminds you "Many people have been at war with themselves. They have not been there for themselves. To see the nature of joy and pain, one must be able to accept oneself and to love and take care of oneself." Be kind to you, embracing the beautiful bundle of creation you are. In doing so, you not only raise your vibration, you lift the world's frequency. Ruth Fishel, author of *Journey Within* said it well with "You will find your strength within you; in places deep where you have not yet dared to visit. Know that you have all that you need to do all that is good and right in your life today."

Dr. Wayne Dyer shared, "The higher self is about serving, loving, and being in a nonjudgmental state of peace." When you embrace yourself –the total experience of your soul, spirit and physical temple, you understand you are love and part of God or whomever you understand or believe to be God. Yes, you are God and that simple awareness brings much relief to humanity's "drama".

This reality is not easily seen. March 2004 marked the first realization of this profound thought for me. During my 10 day Vipassana meditation, I "got" that humanity is composed of something greater than my physical reality. This filtered through my physical temple for years before resurrecting itself again. It is embraced daily as a precious truth.

Invitation to expand:
How would you describe yourself to a blind and deaf person? What do you think of your description? Is it a kind, loving description or the opposite?

I invite you to accept your Divinity and deeply embrace the notion that unconditional love is your birthright. There is no reason to be unhappy. Feel your Divinity pulsating in EVERY cell of your body.

SELF-DISCIPLINE

To accomplish anything in life it is important to discipline your mind and your time. What do you wish to accomplish in life? What is stopping you? Napoleon Hill in *Think and Grow Rich* stated "You either control your mind or it controls your life. Mind control is the result of self-discipline and habit." (Refer to HABITS section for self-disciplining tips).

SELF-IMAGE

Think about what you do daily, the words you use and how you feel. If you took an average of your feelings, what % would be positive, uplifting and what % life draining? According to Maxwell Maltz, "We act, behave and feel according to what we consider our self-image to be and we do not deviate from this pattern."

Zig Ziglar, in *Five Steps to Successful Selling,* offers great advice about building a healthy self-image. His suggestions are below:

1. "Take physical inventory." Understand that physically you are worth millions.
2. "Take mental inventory." Ziglar stated "Make up, dress up and go up." In other words, looking better makes you feel better. Also, listen to teachers and people who make you feel better.
3. "Walk before you can run." In other words, take steps along the way.
4. "Join the smile and compliment club." When you smile and compliment people, you make them and yourself feel better.
5. "Do something for someone else."
6. "Be careful about whom you associate with. Right people will make you feel good. Wrong people can pull you down and make you feel less about yourself."

7. List positive qualities about yourself. These, he says can be developed and extended further.
8. "List past successes."

Zig Ziglar closes by saying, "Nobody on the face of the earth can make you feel inferior without your permission. When you refuse to give others that permission, you'll start accepting yourself. Once you accept yourself, you'll have removed a significant barrier to the growth and success you're capable of attaining."

SELF MASTERY

"Character cannot be built nor anything of value accomplished without self-discipline and that takes courage. It is self -mastery which demonstrates maturity. You will never be truly grown up until you have learned to turn your back on the thing you think you want the most because of something you want more. Most people, in achieving great accomplishments, have first had to do something they did not want to do in order to achieve what they wanted to."
George Romney, 1961 message
entitled *Success The Pursuit of The Difficult*

Reiterating Romney's words, Epictetus expressed, "No man is truly free until he masters himself." Each and every one of you is capable of self-mastery if you commit to pursuing your goals. Focusing on self- discipline will ensure self-mastery.

Kute Blackson, life coach and speaker stated, "I believe that the real security is inside each and every one of us." What will you do with this security- with yourself?

SERVICE

"Service to others is the rent you pay for your room here on earth."
Muhammad Ali

Mahatma Gandhi once stated, "The best way to find yourself is to lose yourself in the service of others." When you serve others, you feel better about yourself and also make a living. Bob Proctor states that you get paid in direct proportion to the amount of service you give. How much service do you give? Is it quality service?

Invitation to expand:
If you abide by the saying As you sow, so shall you reap, you understand integrity is a reflection of service. You serve and are served by everyone you come in contact with. As Earl Nightingale stated "Concern yourself only with your service." Examine your life. Are you happy with your results? If not, brainstorm and on paper, list ways to offer more service. Daily, ask how can you increase your service today and ultimately, increase your rewards?

SILENCE

"Proneness to exaggerate, to suppress or modify the truth, willingly or unwittingly, is a natural weakness of man and silence is necessary in order to surmount it."
Mahatma Gandhi

Silence makes some uncomfortable while others revel in it. Why is that? With all of today's technology, some are unable to silently sit, meditate or seek inner guidance through intuition. Silence is part of life and allows for a deeper understanding of it. Mahatma Gandhi also stated, "It has often occurred to me that a seeker after truth has to be silent. After I practiced silence for some time I saw the spiritual value of it." Silence helps you know yourself and the world better. It sharpens your senses and as Mark Rothko stated "Silence is so accurate."

Silence takes you to the deeper recesses of your soul where no one can travel but yourself. It helps you know you are a whole, magnificent being, capable of anything. Silence helps you appreciate everything and focus on life's abundance and nature's brilliance. Elizabeth Kubler-Ross reminds you, "Learn to get in touch with the silence within yourself and know that

113

everything in this life has a purpose."

SIMPLIFY

"As you simplify your life, the laws of the universe will be simpler; solitude will not be solitude, poverty will not be poverty, nor weakness."
Henry David Thoreau

Invitation to expand:
A practice I enjoy monthly is donating/gifting 3 things I have. This could be clothing no longer worn, something no longer used or that no longer serves me. I do not think of what I can acquire but what can I give? (This paradigm shift may take time to implement). Depending on what the items are, they are disposed of or donated, often to someone I know. Questions I ask include: Have I worn this or used it in the past year? Will I wear it or use it now? If the answer is no- it permanently leaves my home.

In this way, my surroundings are simplified and filled with what I use and love. Energy is allowed to flow and something better replaces the physical and energetic void created. It also helps simplify my mental and soul body as I look around and feel the energy of everything I love.

Perhaps you choose to implement this in your life. Understand, at first you may resist the idea. This is part of the process. As a former 'collector' I resisted and found freedom when I stopped. Work with it and you will find, like everything else, practice makes it easier. It may improve your health on many levels as it is both a physical and energetic clearing.

SOUL

"People talk about mind over matter, the power of the mind. I think the power of the mind is not enough. The next step is soul over matter, the power of the soul. Everyone and everything has a soul. The soul can heal."
Dr. Zhi Gang Sha

What are the characteristics of a soul? In *The Power of Soul,* Dr. Zhi Gang Sha shared, "A human's soul is a golden light being. To see a soul every human must open his/her spiritual eye (Third Eye). The soul can sit in seven main areas or houses. " The 7 areas the soul can sit include: above the genitals; between the genitals and navel; level with the navel; in the heart chakra, throat or head or at the crown chakra."

Dr. Sha also offers sacred practices for developing the soul's power including soul songs and the mantra San San Jiu Lui Ba Yao Wu, Chinese for the sacred healing number 3396815. He suggests repeating this mantra as fast as you can, releasing all attempts of pronouncing it properly.

According to Dr. Sha, the soul has a journey and can be enlightened. A soul's journey equals a spiritual journey. Dr. Sha stated that "Physical life is to serve soul life." He discusses 3 major souls a human has: Tian Ming [(Heaven's Order), Ren Xing (your true nature and self) and Wu Shen (souls of 5 organs: heart (heart shen), spleen (spleen yi), lungs (lung po), kidneys (kidney zhi) and liver (liver hun)]. Each organ, cell, etc. has a soul as does DNA. Dr. Sha ends by stating "The soul journey is the journey to uplift your soul standing in Heaven until it has reached its ultimate destination, which is the realm of the Divine." This journey involves purifying, transforming and enlightening the soul.

Dr. Sha also stated that "Soul enlightenment is a special spiritual standing in Heaven." It involves serving humanity and Gaia well for hundreds of lifetimes; purifying heart, soul and mind and passing spiritual tests. By lifting your soul standing in Heaven, you receive greater blessings including inner peace and joy.

SOUL MATE

"You do not have one soul mate. You have many soul mates in your lifetime that are part of your soul group. More than likely, many of your soul mates are in your life right now or will be in the future. Soul mates can be friends, relatives, husbands, wives, co-workers and lovers. They appear in our lives to teach us and guide us through a variety of different circumstances."
James Van Praagh in his book, *Heaven and Earth*

SOUL INGREDIENTS

During a teleconference on 8 March 2012, Arielle Ford discussed 3 keys to manifesting a soul mate. These 3 keys are: 1) Have "crystal clear clarity." Know who the right person is for you and how you feel with that person. Also, what are the heart traits you desire? 2) "Let go of physical, psychic and emotional clutter." These include memories, trauma, clothing and anything energetically tied to a past relationship. 3) "Feel in EVERY cell of your body that you are worthy." Remember that what you feel, you also attract. The movie *The Secret* left out the feeling part. Be willing to explore the possibility of attracting into your life what you DESIRE. Arielle also suggested doing whatever it takes to THINK and FEEL good.

SPIRIT

"We are not human beings having a spiritual experience. We are spiritual beings having a human experience."
Teilhard de Chardin

What is Spirit?
Spirit is not something external; it is part of your thinking, feeling and actions. According to Dr. Deepak Chopra, "Your true Self is pure, infinite spirit." He also shared that asking what is spirit is like asking Who am I. In The *Path to Love*, Dr. Chopra shared "Attune yourself with spirit and it will speak to you in love. Spirit isn't a phenomenon; it is the whispered truth within a phenomenon. As such, spirit is gentle, it persuades by the softest touch."

Brasilian healer Rubens Faria once stated "We grow in the measure that we understand our spirit; it gives us the sense of love, of compassion, of peace." How do you know when you are open to Spirit? You may have unexpected flashes of joy and feel peaceful. Other signs are smiling often and walking with a bounce to your step.

SPIRITUALITY

"If you don't deal with spiritual malnutrition, you will deal with moral constipation."

PAGONA

Dr. Cornell West in Atlanta, Georgia, 19 January 2010

Wayne Dyer shared "You will build yourself up spiritually by attempting tougher and tougher assignments." For some, these tougher assignments seem everlasting and the question arises when will they end? They end when the lesson is learned. This may take 1 day, 1 week, 1 month, 1 year or 11 years. What may be frustrating is the time the unknown desires to be known. Allowing it to be, as it is, helps you learn the lessons. Resisting may bring you closer to the same assignment repeating.

Judith M. Orloff reminds you that love is an important part of these assignments. She stated, "The bedrock of spirituality is to learn about love." Love is interwoven in the tougher and tougher assignments. Very rewarding on my journey was learning about and embracing self- love. This, for me is a crucial foundation of the spiritual path.

In *Compassion in Action*, Ram Dass stated, "The spiritual journey, as I now conceive of it, is a progression from truth to ever-deepening truth." He shared that he listens and tunes into the deepest truth instead of choosing. What if you tuned into your intuition on your journey? What does it tell you?

A great line in the film *Fight Club* states: "Our great war is our spiritual war. Our great depression is our lives." Your life is a choice and can be transformed. Hearing Dr. Cornell West speak engaged my mind. Moral constipation cannot exist when daily action is directed toward spiritual nutrition.

STILLNESS

"Man is ill because he is never still."
Paracelsus

In *Seven Spiritual Laws of Success*, Dr. Chopra stated "Stillness is the first requirement for manifesting your desires because in your stillness lies your connection to the field of pure potentiality that can orchestrate an infinity of details for you." The stillness within you is a place you may access anytime and anywhere. It is a place of non-judgment and pure awareness with life. Silence is created in the mind when you are still.

Invitation to expand:
Make a daily commitment to be still. Sit in silence in the morning and in the evening. I do this daily and also add gratitude to the experience. Take time to be still with nature, observing the sights, sounds and scents around you. Finally, practice non-judgment beginning each day with "Today, I shall judge nothing that occurs."

STRESS

"Any time one person makes an effort to contact a deeper part of him or herself, balance his or her emotions, and deflect the stress momentum, others benefit. As more individuals learn to maintain their poise and balance and refrain from adding to the incoherence around them, they help to counterbalance the frequency of stress."
Doc Childre and Howard Martin

A Chinese Proverb states "Tension is who you think you should be. Relaxation is who you are." Everything is made of energy and different energy states resonate at different frequencies. The frequency of stress is lower than the frequency of love. Frederick Saunders reminded you that "Brain cells create ideas. Stress kills brain cells. Stress is not a good idea." Although it may sound comical, Saunders' quote is full of wisdom. How many times do you attempt to generate ideas while stressed? What is the outcome?

What is your passion? What are your gifts? Did you discover them? If not, what are you waiting for? Pavel Stoyanov shared "The major cause of stress is the inability of people to discover their real nature. Discover your gifts, follow them and you will never feel stressed."

SUCCESS

"Success comes from the initiative and following up...persisting, eloquently expressing the depth of your love. What simple action could you take today to produce a new momentum toward success in your life?"
Anthony Robbins

"Success is the progressive realization of a worthy ideal." Earl Nightingale came up with this definition of success in 1951 and Bob Proctor has used it since. Proctor reminds you an ideal is something you trade your life for. It is worthy of you and something you must be passionate about because you trade your time for it. It also must be something you see yourself accomplishing no matter what the obstacles appear to be. Progressive means you are working toward your goal. Albert Schweitzer shared that "Success is not the key to happiness. Happiness is the key to success. If you love what you are doing, you will be successful."

While there are many interpretations to the acronym SUCCESS, a favorite is found on http://ezinearticles.com/?updates=Bradley_Buller. According to Bradley Buller, 7 Secrets Of Success exist and are summarized by 7 letters in **SUCCESS. SUCCESS** stands for:

S for Solo focus. Identify and work toward your goal.

U for Undying conviction, leadership and imagination.

C for Crystal Clear Path. Know exactly where you are headed.

C for Connection to The Heart. You must LOVE what you do. It must be something that if you don't do it you will literally stop living and breathing. This must be one of the most important things in your life. Use your brain to think but use your heart to drive you.

E for Extraordinary Energy. Have enthusiasm and look forward to getting up in the morning to begin work.

S for Skill Set. This refers to your communication skills.

S for Stop at Nothing. Do whatever it takes, not allowing negativity in.

Also, remember everything is about attitude. With a positive attitude you succeed. With a negative one, you will not.

Invitation to expand:
How do YOU define success? How do you spend your time? What are you willing to trade your life for? Examine what makes you happy and get to work on it. Remember Michael Jordan's words "I missed more than 9,000 shots in my career. I lost almost 300 games. On 26 occasions I have been entrusted to take the game winning shot... and missed. I failed over and over and over again in my life and that is precisely why I succeed."

SOUL INGREDIENTS

SUNLIGHT

"If we could convert 0.03 percent of the sunlight that falls on the earth into energy, we could meet all of our projected needs for 2030."
Ray Kurzweil

Dr. F. Batmanghelidj stated, "To asthmatics, sunlight is medicine. Light from the sun acts on cholesterol deposits on the skin and converts them to vitamin D." The sun can be used to heal the mind, body and spirit. This is discussed at www.solarhealing.com and an example of Hira Ratan Manek (HRM) is given. He claimed better physical, mental, emotional and spiritual health after sun gazing.

HRM, among others, proved a person can live just on solar energy for long periods without eating. This is known as the HRM phenomenon and is used to cure psychosomatic, mental and physical illnesses and increase memory and mental strength. After practicing HRM for 3 months, one's psychological problems can disappear and confidence and a balanced mind develop, overcoming fear and life's problems. After 6 months of practice, one is said to be free from physical illness.

According to HRM, "Sun energy is the source that powers the brain, which can enter and leave the human body or brain through one organ- the human eye. Eyes are the Sun Energy's entry door to the human brain and are also known as the windows of the soul." Recent research found that the eye has many functions other than vision. The eyes are complex organs with 5 billion parts, more than a spacecraft (with 6-7 million parts). HRM asserts the rainbow is in the eye and the sun's seven colors are only the reflection found in the eye. You can create a rainbow by being in the garden and observing water flowing beneath as the sun moves above.

TAO TE CHING

The *Tao Te Ching* is "The Classic of the Way and Its Virtue" written by Lao Tzu thousands of years ago. As a world literature classic, it had a huge impact on Asian thought. Lao Tzu or the "Old Master" teaches you the Tao or Way of everything. It is useful in business leadership, harmony and daily balance and as an embodiment of humility, generosity and spontaneity.

TEACH/TEACHERS/TEACHING

"If you think in terms of a year, plant a seed; if in terms of ten years, plant trees; if in terms of 100 years, teach the people."
Confucius

Aristotle shared, "Teaching is the highest form of understanding." Everyone is both a student and teacher many times in life. When you are a student you have much to learn. When you master that understanding, you can teach it. While teaching, you help others learn or discover new things and you also learn. Mark Van Doren stated "The art of teaching is the art of assisting discovery."

I was blessed to serve as adjunct faculty teaching World Cultures. In this role, I was both a facilitator in discovery and a student, understanding self and others, particularly first year college students. Two lessons I learned were to always remain open to wisdom and opinions from wherever they arrive and treat all students as geniuses. Not only will they look at you funny, some may embrace their innate genius and transform their life. To witness this is extremely powerful. Once learning stops, it is time for continued renewal and thirst for more knowledge, otherwise comfort, old habits and stagnation linger.

What concepts, if taught, would change the world? Lao Tzu stated it well with "I have just three things to teach: simplicity, patience, compassion. These three are your greatest treasures. "As teachers, educators, professors, what do you teach? What seeds do you plant in your school, home and community? What fruits do you seek? Do you enjoy the labors of your harvest?

THOUGHTS/THINKING

"Don't think of anything you don't want. Spend time focusing on what you want."
Bob Proctor

SOUL INGREDIENTS

Bob Proctor studied and continues to study the mind for over 50 years. If you have an opportunity to hear him speak, I highly recommend it. He speaks about many things including the power of thoughts. If you put positive information in, you get positive thoughts out. However, you receive negative thoughts if you put negative thoughts in. Alfred A. Montapert reiterates this by stating "Every time you get angry, you poison your own system."

Donald Trump gave the following advice "As long as you're going to think anyway, think big." William James, a psychologist, philosopher and author who passed away in 1910, spoke about the perception of thinking. He stated, "Many people think they are thinking when they are merely rearranging their prejudices."

James Allen, author of *As A Man Thinketh* stated, "You are today where your thoughts have brought you. You will be tomorrow where your thoughts take you." Look around you. Where have your thoughts taken you? What you think reflects what you focus on and choose to see. If you are in the right environment at the right time, with the right people and the right thoughts with the right reasons (as Napoleon Hill stated in *Think and Grow Rich*), you'll get the right results. Do you realize when you change your thoughts, your world changes?

"Keep your thoughts positive
because your thoughts become your words.
Keep your words positive
because your words become your behaviors.
Keep your behaviors positive
because your behaviors become your habits
Keep your habits positive
because your habits become your values.
Keep your values positive
because your values become your destiny."
Mahatma Gandhi

The Upanishads mirror Gandhi's words. They state "Watch your thoughts; they become words. Watch your words; they become actions. Watch your actions; they become habits. Watch your habits; they become character. Watch your character; for it becomes your destiny." Reread and study these words. Let them sink in. Understand and embrace them. Do whatever you need to do to watch your thoughts. Guard them as if your life depended on it for it does. Mike Dooley, author of *Infinite Possibilities,* reiterates this stating, "Your thought become things. Your thoughts are the only reason anything has happened or not happened in your life."

Dr. Raymond Holliwell, in *Working with the Law,* spoke of abundance. He shared that a consciousness that does not embrace abundance cannot see it. In other words, if collective consciousness or individual consciousness does not allow/acknowledge/open their mind(s) to it, it is not seen or thought and therefore remains impossible. He stated, "All the poverty in the world arises from a poverty consciousness, whether collective or individual. There is more food in the air undiscovered than we can use. There is more power in a single drop of water or in a lump of sugar than man can realize at this moment. The supply is greater than the demand and the demand is determined by man's own thinking."

TODAY I WILL

In *The Greatest Salesman in The World,* Og Mandino listed 10 great statements to commit to today. They are as follows:

> "Today I will begin a new life.
> Today I will greet this day with love in my heart.
> Today I will persist until I succeed.
> I am nature's greatest miracle.
> I will live this day as if it is my last.
> Today I will be master of my emotions.
> I will laugh at the world.
> Today I will multiply my value a hundred fold.
> I will act now.
> I will pray."

What WILL you choose to do today? Will you release the energy of love, peace and harmony? Will you be the light and allow your light to shine?

TRAVEL

"The real meaning of travel, like that of a conversation by the fireside, is the discovery of oneself through contact with other people and its condition is self-commitment in the dialogue."
Dr. Paul Tournier

Travel is a precious, eye opening gift of understanding; compassion; patience; vulnerability; Unity and Truth. It enables one to see beyond human eyes and taste life's kaleidoscope. I often say "Travel gave me new eyes, new ears, a new mouth and a new heart. It has inspired me like nothing else."

It often amazes me the number of people who desire to travel yet allow fear and other illusions to stop them. Often, I suggest they make the decision and everything will fall into place for the trip. This doesn't sit well with many.

On the other hand, others, like me, are fearless and take any and every opportunity to explore the world; its fascinating people; food; history and culture. For the experience of visiting 28 countries, I remain a grateful, inquisitive adventurer, exploring and embracing humanity.

Invitation to expand:
If you were to travel anywhere and left tomorrow, where would you go? Why? What 3 things would you bring with you? What is stopping you from going (besides yourself)?

TRUTH

"Not everything you see is real, not everything you don't see is false." Pagona

As I observed my Latina neighbor, I understood her limitations and fears stopped her from befriending me. She was caught up in what many on the planet are caught in. What is this? Her view of me was limited based on what she saw- a white woman speaking like any other 'white' woman in

America. My attempts at friendliness were met by a flat hello while her 4 yr. old daughter smiled and gravitated toward me as her mom pulled her away with the words Mind your business. Thus came the above insight, "Not everything you see is real and not everything you don't see is false."

Many times people are surprised to hear I am a Greek American woman who fluently speaks another language with immigrant parents who speak broken English. They hear an educated Caucasian woman speak English without an apparent accent. They are amazed that I traveled to their homeland and hold a deep inner understanding of cultural challenges. My truth is intertwined with what I choose to expose myself to; world cultures; people of different faiths and theories; all catalysts for intimate conversations with supposed 'strangers.'

"All truth passes through three phases: First, it is ridiculed. Second, it is violently opposed. Third, it is accepted as self-evident."
Arthur Schopenhauer, 1788-1860

What is truth? Mahatma Gandhi answered this question with "What is Truth? A difficult question; but I solved it for myself by saying that it is what the "voice within" tells you." In other words, truth is your intuition. Are you listening?

Karen Sawyer, in her book, *The Dangerous Man,* wrote "I have come to realize the accepted version of 'the truth' is often a façade for another, often secret agenda. A secret isn't 'sinister' –it only becomes when you keep that knowledge to yourself to manipulate and control others." Think about what you view as truth and why you view it as such. Could another possibility exist-another version of truth? If so, are you open to it? Dr. Cornell West stated "We have got to attempt to tell the truth and that truth is painful. It is a truth that is against the thick lies of mainstream."

Invitation to expand:
Whitney Otto stated "When someone tells you the truth, lets you think for yourself, experiences your own emotions; he's treating you as if you are a true equal, as a friend." Seek out people who are truth seekers and tell the truth. You live in the truth of your understanding, what you consider the truth. However, in your daily interactions with others, you often hear a contradictory

view-other people's truth. Are you willing to hear and understand someone else's truth if you do not agree with it? If so, what can you learn from it? Is this truth a reflection of you?

The opposite of worry is UNDERSTANDING

"Tell me and I'll forget; show me and I might remember; involve me and I'll understand."
Mike Lambert, acupuncturist, psychologist
and former Health and Safety investigator

What happens when you do not understand something or someone? Oftentimes, this person or thing that appears foreign is ridiculed. Bob Proctor states "If you operate from not knowing, thoughts go to worry and doubt. The opposite of worry is understanding." When you have faith and trust that all unfolds as it should at the right time, right place, under the right conditions, there is no place for worry and doubt.

Invitation to expand:
What needs understanding now in your life? What steps can you take for a deeper understanding of self and thus a greater understanding of another?

UNIFIED FIELD

David Lynch, in *Catching the Big Fish* does an excellent job describing what physics call the Unified Field:
"Ideas are like fish. If you want to catch little fish, you can stay in the shallow water. If you want to catch big fish, you got to go deeper.
Down deep, the fish are more powerful and more pure. They are hungry and abstract. There are all kinds of fish swimming down there. There are fish for business, fish for sports. There are fish for everything.
Everything, anything that is a thing, comes up from the deepest level. Modern physics calls that level the Unified Field. The more your consciousness, your awareness is expanded, the deeper you go toward this source and the

bigger the fish you catch."

UNIVERSAL LAWS

"The Laws of the Universe don't change, our awareness changes."
Mary Morrissey

In Raymond Holliwell's book, *Working with the Law,* the following 11 Universal Laws are described: **1) The Law of Thinking 2) The Law of Supply 3) The Law of Attraction 4) The Law of Receiving 5) The Law of Increase 6) The Law of Compensation 7) The Law of Non- Resistance 8) The Law of Forgiveness 9) The Law of Sacrifice 10) The Law of Obedience 11) The Law of Success.**

Each law is real and operates continuously, independent of your awareness. Successful people including two of my mentors, Bob Proctor and Mary Morrissey study and apply these Laws. If you do nothing else, continuously reread, study and apply these principles. As Holliwell stated, "It is the realization of The Law in action that determines manifestation." Each law is simplified below using Holliwell's words:

The Law of Thinking can be simplified with Holliwell's' words: "We are what we are according to our state of thinking. We attract only what we think or create." We attract the energy of the thought-whether positive or negative.

The Law of Supply, according to Dr. Raymond Holliwell is summed up with "Man possesses the whole world and all its wealth, yet is only able to enjoy what his consciousness permits him to discern." If you think and operate from a space of there is enough food, cash, etc., or conversely, there is not enough, your life will respond accordingly.

Dr. Raymond Holliwell stated that **The Law of Attraction** works "When you constantly expect that which you persistently desire. Desire connects you with the thing desired and expectation draws it into your life." For the Law of Attraction to work, desire and expectation must exist. Expect and desire the best!

The Law of Receiving states: "We are continually drawing into life what we give and expect. Whether we attract good or bad, it is governed by the same principle." Dr. Raymond Holliwell

127

The **Law of Increase** works, as Holliwell stated, "When man praises, he lifts his consciousness to a higher realm and becomes a greater channel to receive the good that is ever waiting to come to him."

The **Law of Compensation**, according to Holliwell, states: "You must earn what you receive or you cannot keep it." 3 things hinder this law: Do you expect something for nothing? Do you look for cheap items (items of value have a higher vibration and can be used instead of cheap) and do you hate to pay bills?

Law of Non-Resistance, according to Holliwell, works when you: "Remove and dissolve every obstacle by blessing it and being willing to understand it." In other words, do not worry, complain or do anything that resists good coming to you.

The **Law of Forgiveness**, according to Holliwell, states: "Only when we forgive are we forgiven." If you cut off the weeds in your garden, they may be temporarily gone yet will sprout again. They must be completely pulled out.

The **Law of Sacrifice,** according to Holliwell, requires that "Something always has to be paid for something else."

The **Law of Obedience** speaks about obeying the Law of Truth and doing what is right. To obey this law, Holliwell suggests: "Live in the present, do your highest duty every day, forget the past and let the future take care of itself."

The **Law of Success**, according to Holliwell, states that you can succeed if you "Know you can succeed and proceed to think, live and act in that strong conviction." The key is to have an "I can" attitude.

UPPER LIMIT PROBLEM (UPL)

According to Gay Hendricks, Ph.D., you have an upper limit problem. "Each of us has a thermostat that determines how much love, creativity and success we allow ourselves to enjoy. When you exceed the inner thermostat setting, you often do something to sabotage yourself, causing you to drop back into the old, familiar zone where you feel secure."

Invitation to expand:
Now that you are aware of the UPL, what changes do you choose to embrace? How do you observe the so called 'obstacles' in your life? Will you

acknowledge you are responsible for you and may be the biggest thing in your way?

VIBRATION

"Hard work is not the path to Well- Being. Feeling good is the path to Well-Being. You don't create through action; you create through vibration. Then, your vibration calls action from you."
Abraham Hicks

Did you know how you say things may create resistance to receiving that into your life? Abraham Hicks stated "When you talk about what you want and why you want it, there's usually less resistance within you than when you talk about what you want and how you're going to get it. When you pose questions you don't have answers for, like how, where, when, who, it sets up a contradictory vibration that slows everything down." Words, like everything have energy and vibrate at certain frequencies. The more loving, supportive and compassionate your words, the higher the frequencies they vibrate in. (This is evident in the Water section).

You are all energy and everything in the Universe is made of energy. Be mindful of the thoughts you choose. Your thoughts, like everything else vibrate at a certain frequency and can be life depleting or life affirming. John Assaraf and Murray Smith, authors of *The Answers* share "Every thought you form broadcasts a distinct and particular frequency and that frequency elicits a response from the quantum universe as surely as a swinging hammer has an impact on the surface it strikes." What frequency are you broadcasting?

We spoke about the importance of love in life and in awareness. Dr. Wayne Dyer, in his book, *The Power of Intention* speaks about the vibration of love. He stated, "One individual who lives and vibrates to the energy of pure love and reverence for all of life will counterbalance the negativity of 750,000 individuals who calibrate at the lower weakening levels." Imagine the global implications of millions of people vibrating at the frequency of love and negating millions more of a lower frequency. Being aware of this may cause enough thinking to stop you from engaging from a place other than love.

VISUALIZATION

"Visualization is like a language you can use to talk to your subconscious. It is a universal language for people that don't speak your language."
Jon Gabriel, author and weight loss expert

Andy Baggott, in his book *Blissology: The Art and Science of Happiness*, mentioned 4 exercises to help with visualization. He tells you to focus on something familiar and move to objects and then people and finally, to see yourself.

Baggott suggests that to imagine something familiar, imagine a room like a kitchen. See the color of the wall, the view from the window, etc. When imagining an object, imagine a simple object, like a box. Notice the size, color and what it is made from. Move to a more complex object like a house, walking through it noticing everything including what you feel. When imagining people, imagine and visualize your closest friend doing a daily activity like cooking. What is he/she wearing, what is the location? Next, imagine yourself in front of a mirror. Notice your expression, clothes and environment. Imagine walking down your street and imagine yourself doing something extraordinary. What are you imagining? How does that make you feel?

Louise L. Hay, founder of Hay House, offers a wonderful visualization practice. Hay suggested looking in the mirror two times a day for 30 days affirming out loud "I accept myself unconditionally right now." Try this and remember Anthony Robbins words "Whatever you hold in your mind on a consistent basis is exactly what you'll experience in your life."

WISDOM

John C. Maxwell stated "99% of everything in life I don't need to know about. Focus on 1% that gives the highest return." What if you focused on the 1 %, what would your life look like? How would this change your habits, your thoughts, and your life?

In his book, *The Breakthrough Experience,* Dr. John F. Demartini lists the following 10 Daily Pillars of Wisdom:

1) Inspired Action	2) Loving Service
3) Grateful Prayer	4) Divine Guidance
5) Sharing Wisdom	6) Caring Sincerely
7) Silent Presence	8) Studying Truths
9) Temperature Rhythm	10) Fair Exchange

How can you incorporate Demartini's wisdom into your life?

Invitation to expand:
A Greek proverb states "Wonder is the beginning of wisdom." What if you examined what you wonder about and shared this with a friend? What if, for 1 week, you lovingly took action on 1 of Dr. Demartini's pillars, practiced daily and recorded the results? For example, what if you chose grateful prayer? Instead of thinking how upset you are with your child, brother, father, husband, mother, sister or wife, you give thanks for this person's presence in your life and wish the best possible for him/her?

WHAT GAVE YOU THE GREATEST WISDOM? What would occur if you shared that wisdom with another and then another?

THE POWER OF ILLUMINATED WORDS

"To speak ill of anyone is to speak ill of yourself."
Afghan Proverb

The power of the spoken and written word is tremendous. A Vietnamese saying states "It doesn't cost anything to have loving speech." Words inspire, heal and have the potential to inflict psychological pain and wounds. When speaking, speak well of others, as how you speak of others is how you speak of yourself.

I once heard T. Harv Eker state, "How you do anything is how you do everything." How do you think about another? What words do you use? Perhaps reflecting on this will motivate your mind and mouth to use positive, life affirming and empowering words about self and others. Perhaps it will cause reflective thinking about how you do the little things.

Rudyard Kipling, who lived between 1865- 1936 stated: "I am by nature a dealer in words and words are the most powerful drug known to humanity."

Dr. Richard Bartlett, ND & DC in his book *The Physics of Miracles,* stated, "Words are a cup of light that contain holographic patterns and pictures." He also shared that as auditory and conceptual templates, words can unlock what you focus on. What words are you using?

Although using words to describe spiritual phenomenon and feelings may be difficult, words are what you have. What words will define how you choose to speak about you, your life, your choices, your surroundings and everything in you?

What words will you pass on to children and future generations? What words will dictate your choices? Which words do you tell yourself every am and pm? Which words do you define health, wealth and your relationships by? Which words do you empower yourself with?

Choose positive, life affirming and empowering words. As the late Dr. David Simon taught, before a word is uttered from your lips, ask yourself: "Is it true? Is it necessary? Is it kind?"

I like to say "Think carefully about the power of your words for they are like the oxygen you breathe in and the carbon dioxide you breathe out. Words come from thought and deplete your qi or make great deposits to your longevity and health, 365 days a year."

Invitation to expand:

Ivan Petrovich Pavlov stated, "Words act as stimulants and this is why they can provoke reactions in the body." A young man, whom my nephew and I met on a plane, shared the power of words with me. After sharing pieces of his life, I asked a question to which he replied that Neale Donald Walsch's book, *Conversations With God*, stopped him from taking his life. This, my dear friends is the power of the written and spoken word. Use it carefully.

In your mind, peruse all the books you read and the inspiring conversations you engaged in. Think about the power of each word, of those that inspired you and changed your life. Embrace positive words, people and experiences. Speak and breathe compassion and love.

WORRY

"It makes no sense to worry about things you have no control over because there's nothing you can do about them, and why worry about things you do control? The activity of worrying keeps you immobilized."
Wayne Dyer

What if you understood the physiological effects of worry? Would this prevent you from doing it? Perhaps it would decrease it? Charles W. May stated, "Worry affects the circulation, the heart, the glands and the whole nervous system and profoundly affects health." Worry tells the Universe you lack faith and must engage in the habit of 'worry' instead.

Worry is like attempting to drive yet your foot constantly clamps on the brake. Worry immobilizes you into a state of 'stuckness' and as a paradigm, repeats as regularly as you breathe. It takes conscious effort to stop and when you do, it propels you forward into an ever expanding space of possibility.

Peggy McColl, in her book *Your Destiny Switch*, offers insight about why people worry. She states you worry because you are: afraid of something; afraid to release anger; you are not appreciating what is working; you don't enjoy the present situation; you lost faith; you forgot about your strengths and gifts or you hold false beliefs. To replace worry, McColl states you may wish to feel calm, confident and believe. Also helpful are: infusing humor; using a verbal cue like "That's enough of that"; engaging in a physical activity like jumping jacks; helping someone else; listening to positive music or asking "What would I like to experience?"

YOU

You look to others for many things including love, appreciation, approval and advice. What if you embraced Mary Morrissey's words "You are the highest authority on the path you should take." How would your life change if you looked to you for your answers, instead of looking to others? What if you listened to your intuition to answer the questions of your soul?

In the film, *The Answer is You,* Rev. Michael B. Beckwith mentioned that "You create your environment from within yourself." What you think and do comes from you and your surroundings. In *Book III of Conversations with God*, Neale Donald Walsch states "Who you are is love. Love is unlimited, eternal and free. Therefore, you are unlimited, eternal, and free by nature." As human beings, you decide what you are being. Your experience is based on your perceptions which are based on your understanding.

As my friend Nancy Cosgray told me in 2009 "Work on you, when you do, you work on the world." These words resonated with me then and continue to today. What if, instead of "What can I get"? you ask "What can I give?" What if, instead of asking, "Why is he/she not returning my calls"? ask, "Why am I devoting so much time to thinking about my calls"? As stated earlier, to question is important but more important is asking a better question for the question will guide the answers you receive.

ZEN

"When you really laugh, suddenly mind disappears. The whole Zen methodology is how to get into no-mind -- laughter is one of the beautiful doors to get to it. As far as I know, dancing and laughter are the best, natural, easily approachable doors."
Osho

According to *Zen Around the World*, written by Annellen M. Simpkins and C. Alexander Simpkins, "the interweaving of three influences-Yoga, Taoism and Buddhism, helped create modern Zen." Zen began in India and Tibet and flowed into Europe and North America. Zen was spoken about in *The Upanishads*- the Indian philosophical writings sacred to the Hindus. R. H Blyth stated it well with the metaphor: "India was the woman, China the man and Zen the wonderful child."

John Bradshaw stated, "Children are natural Zen masters; their world is brand new in each and every moment." Watch children while they play and interact with others, they are always present to the now. For them, the past doesn't exist and neither does the future.

AMAKAZE

According to Wendy Esko, author of *Introducing Macrobiotic Cooking,* amazake is made from rice and koji (rice culture). Koji is added to steamed sweet rice and fermented for 8-20 hours. Amazake is low in fat, high in fiber and contains complex carbohydrates, B vitamins and niacin. It is extremely good for the digestion and is traditionally used in Japan to treat digestive issues in adults and children.

CACAO- FAGITO TOUS THEOUS
(FOOD OF THE GODS)

According to Lindsey Duncan, ND, DC of www.drlindsey.com, cacao (Theobroma cacao), or "food of the gods", is the purest form of chocolate. It is a superfood with a rich history and many health benefits.

The ancient Olmec, Mayan and Aztec cultures consumed cacao regularly. They also held it in high esteem as they included it in religious, medical, economic and cultural life. Its many health benefits include: supporting heart health, energy levels, free radical scavenging, positive mood and increased focus. It is high in antioxidants and contains the feel good chemical anandamide and the chemical theobromine which boosts energy.

"CAFFEINE IS A DRUG"

In his book, *Integrative Nutrition*, NY's Integrative Nutrition (IIN) founder Joshua Rosenthal states "Millions of Americans jump-start their days with a cup of coffee and drink another cup or two or three throughout the day. Starbucks stores and others proliferated throughout the country and the world. More people try to move faster and faster to keep pace with the increasing demands of modern society. Coffee represents 75% of all caffeine consumed in the United States. If sugar is America's number one addiction, then coffee ranks a close second. Caffeine is a drug and we are a nation of drug addicts."

In his book, *Caffeine Blues*, Stephen Cherniske, M.S., Research and Clinical Nutritionist, states that caffeine affects your body and mind and is addictive. According to Cherniske, caffeine affects your body by: 1) Causing the liver to breakdown coffee which is absorbed at once by every organ and tissue and crosses the blood brain barrier. 2) Blocking adenosine receptors which cause neurons to continually fire making you feel alert. 3) Activating stress response caused by epinephrine and norepinephrine pushed out by the adrenal glands. 4) Elevating stress hormone cortisol (with daily caffeine) so that sleep quality decreases and immune system is affected. 5) Triggering dopamine release, a neurotransmitter affecting our feelings and producing a 'high'. 6) Contributing to deficiency of DHEA (the vitality hormone) caused by elevated cortisol. DHEA is the precursor to estrogen and testosterone and thus affects immunity and aging. 7) Contributing to malnutrition as caffeine and possibly other ingredients in coffee and soft drinks cause increased loss of thiamine, Vitamin B, calcium and other minerals in urine.

Cherniske states that the mental and emotional effects of caffeine may make anxiety worse and contribute to anxiety and panic in panic disorder patients. Also, caffeine may aggravate PMS and those drinking large amounts of caffeine may experience withdrawal symptoms after stopping consumption.

In the documentary *Hungry for a Change*, the implication of many foods is discussed including soda and diet soda. Dr. Mercola stated, "Most pilots are aware of diet soda because it is well recognized within the pilot association that you don't drink this because it can cause severe aberrations in your vision that will potentially lead to problems with your flying." In the same documentary, Dr. Christiane Winthrop, best- selling Women's health author, stated "Aspartame (an ingredient in diet soda) + caffeine create excitotoxin that kills brain cells. Before they die, you have an excitement like buzz. Females do it as a way to keep weight down, they don't eat and have next buzz of diet cola."

Invitation to expand:

While 1 cup of coffee or soda/day may not be as detrimental to health as many, the cumulative effects may be hazardous. What shall you do? Try herbal tea or an herbal coffee alternative like Teeccino Caffé Inc., www.teeccino.com. This caffeine free beverage is brewed like coffee and available in 7 flavors with ingredients like roasted carob, barley and chicory root. Also available is an instant coffee substitute from Kaffree Roma Roasted Grain www.wfds.com, also made from barley and chicory.

In lieu of soda, try adding a drop of essential oil (lemon, lime, grapefruit) to your water or add fresh squeezed lemon, lime or tangerine juice. Also, make fresh vegetable juices or fresh fruit juices. Experiment with different vegetable juices, adding fruits to sweeten.

CHAMOMILE

Growing up in a traditional Greek home, I drank chamomile and use it often. Chamomile is an herb from a flowering plant in the daisy family. In Greece it grows wild. The fresh and dried flowers are used to make tea.

According to www.homeremediesweb.com, chamomile contains the essential oil, bisabolol, which is anti-irritant, anti-inflammatory and anti-microbial. Chamomile aids in many conditions including: sleep disorders; anxiety and panic attacks; wounds; burns and scrapes; skin conditions such as psoriasis; eczema; chickenpox; diaper rash and stomach problems including menstrual cramps and stomach flu. It is considered a home remedy for stomach cramps (as it is said to be antispasmodic) and Irritable Bowel Syndrome (IBS).

If you are on blood thinners or are allergic to plants in the same family (daisy, marigold and chrysanthemum), you may wish to avoid camomile. Also, it should be avoided in pregnancy because it may stimulate the uterus.

CHIA SEEDS- MAYAN SUPERFOOD

According to alternative health specialist and celebrity nutritionist, Lindsey Duncan ND, CN of www.dr.lindsey.com, chia seeds were a main part of the Aztec and Mayan diet. They consumed chia regularly, grinding it into flour, pressing it for oil and mixing it with water. They used chia to stimulate saliva flow and relieve joint pain. Chia was also thought to increase energy and stamina. It received its name from the Mayan word for "strength."

Chia seeds deliver maximum nutrients with minimum calories. They are rich in fiber (about 11 grams/ounce), omega fatty acids, calcium, antioxidants, protein, iron, copper, niacin and zinc. According to Dr. Duncan, "chia absorbs up to 12 times its own weight and expands to curb appetite."

CINNAMON

Kathi Keville, director of the American Herb Association and editor of the American Herb Association Quarterly newsletter and aromatherapy and herb teacher for over 25 years speaks about cinnamon's therapeutic uses.

Keville states that cinnamon's scent stirs the appetite, invigorates and warms the senses and may produce a joyful feeling. Cinnamon oil can be distilled from the leaf or bark. Cinnamon bark is 40-50 % cinnamaldehyde and 4-10 % eugenol and the leaf is 3 % cinnamaldehyde and 70-90 % eugenol.

Cinnamon's therapeutic properties include: antiseptic, digestive, antiviral and topically it relieves muscle spasms and rheumatic pain. It is generally used as a physical and emotional stimulant. Researchers found it reduces drowsiness, irritability and headache pain. As a liniment (8 drops/ounce), it increases circulation and sweating.

Precautions for cinnamon include not using more than ½ drop in the bath and avoiding it in cosmetics because it may redden and burn skin. Both the bark and leaf oils can irritate mucous membranes.

COCONUT OIL

Coconut oil, in its unrefined, unfiltered; hexane free state is beneficial for numerous things. It is used globally in cooking and as a face and hair moisturizer. *Note- it may stain clothing, sheets or pillows.

Below are 33 uses for coconut oil, courtesy of The Seed Lady of Watts, who compiled this over 20 years ago. List obtained on www.Nutiva.com.

1. Eat 1 spoonful when you need an energy boost.

2. Take 1 spoonful with your vitamins to help improve absorption.
3. Replace unhealthy vegetable oils in cooking/baking with coconut oil.
4. Add 1 spoonful to your smoothies for extra nutrition and flavor.
5. Eat 1 spoonful with each meal to improve digestion.
6. Take up to 5 spoonfuls a day for improved thyroid function.
7. Use as a base for homemade chocolate candy.
8. Use to condition wooden cutting boards.
9. Use as a super conditioner on your hair (apply to dry hair, leave in as long as possible and shampoo as usual).
10. Rub a tiny amount on your palms, apply to hair and style.
11. Keep a small container in purse for lip moisturizer.
12. *Use as a face and/or body moisturizer, rub until fully absorbed.
13. Add 1 spoonful to your dog or cat's food.
14. Use instead of shaving cream.
15. Use as the base for a homemade body scrub.
16. Add to bath tub as moisturizing soak.
17. Soothes chicken pox, shingles and skin rashes or irritations.
18. Use to treat athlete's foot, ringworm, fungal or yeast infections.
19. Spread a thin layer on cuts or burns to speed up healing.
20. Use on delicate tissue around eyes to help prevent wrinkles.
21. Use to remove stuck gum from your hair.
22. Use in place of massage oil.
23. Use on your baby's diaper rash.
24. Use to help reduce visibility of stretch marks or prevent them.
25. Nursing moms, use on nipples to prevent cracking and irritation.
26. Consuming coconut oil may increase milk flow for nursing moms.
27. Use to relieve yeast infections, dryness and discomfort.
28. Apply to bee stings or bug bites to soothe and heal.
29. For nosebleeds, coat inside of nostrils with coconut oil regularly.
30. Helps soothe/heal hemorrhoids.
31. Use a spoonful to help with heartburn, acid reflux or indigestion.
32. Mix with peppermint, lemon balm, rosemary, or tea tree essential oil to make an excellent insect repellant.
33. Helps detox the body during a cleanse or fast.

COCONUT WATER:
NATURE'S ELECTROLYTE SOURCE

Coconut water is one of nature's healthiest, nutritious beverages. In its natural state, it is free of sugar and full of electrolytes (salts, specifically ions your cells use to carry electrical impulses to other cells). In *Food Energetics: The Spiritual, Emotional and Nutritional Power of What We Eat,* Steve Gagné stated "Foods from coconuts are supportive to kidney and renal functions. Coconuts (milk, water and kernel) can help with regulation of minerals and sodium levels and assist in the maintenance of urinary tract health by helping reduce infections."

Since electrolytes need to be replaced, coconut water offers a sugar and chemical free natural solution. For optimal nutrition, opening a fresh coconut and drinking its water is best. If this is not feasible, coconut water in bottles or cartons is better than that in aluminum cans.

COOKING

"Cooking is alchemy in daily life. It is a transformation of energy that requires the ability to organize and manipulate the elements of fire, water, air and earth. Cooking is the highest development of an art. It is an art that creates and sustains life as well as one that celebrates it as do painting, drama, literature, music and dance."
Saul Miller

How many dread cooking or complain that you do not know how? Cooking is beautiful and a welcoming part of my day. On the other hand, one of my sisters does not enjoy it. Why? She feels she is not good at it. It takes practice for some while for others it is like second nature. Experiment with simple recipes first and then without. Some of the best chefs do not use recipes. However, for baking, recipes are essential. Let go of any fear surrounding how the food will turn out.

The important thing for you who classify yourselves as not good cooks is to change your paradigm about cooking or find someone who is a good cook. Perhaps barter for cooking in exchange for your greatest skills. Also, nutritious smoothies; fresh vegetable juice and raw food can be prepared that require no cooking. All are quick and nutrient rich alternatives to a cooked meal. As Harriet Van Horne stated in Vogue in October 1956, "Cooking is like love, it should be entered into with abandon or not at all."

EGGS
(use organic, ideally from local organic farm)

Eggs are a great source of protein, cholesterol and choline (one of the B Vitamins that helps reduce inflammation). Ensure that the eggs are organic, free range and ideally from a local farmer. Bright orange yolks indicate eggs are from free range chickens.

What may surprise you is that in Russia, eggs are highly regarded and used in traditional healing. According to Alla Svirinskaya, author of *Energy Secrets,* most Russian households display a wooden or painted egg. Alla shares that for Russians, "Eggs symbolize newborn life, development and growth." She also states "Eggs stand for purity; buried within the egg lies the potential for true divine power."

In addition to eggs symbolizing the beginning of life, Alla states that eggs are highly effective at absorbing spiritual and psychic negativity. She offers an egg bedtime ritual for disturbed sleep or repeatedly dreaming of the same person. Write your name on an egg in pen or pencil and place it on your bedside table, level with your head. Let it remain there for 7 days. If it cracks (it absorbed too much negative energy) throw it away and replace it with another. Throw it away after 7 days.

In his book, *Food Energetics: The Spiritual, Emotional and Nutritional Power of What We Eat,* Steve Gagné stated eggs have an ability to bind and hold and when eaten in excess can manifest as cravings for sweets, coffee and spicy foods. He shared that "The individual who eats a lot of eggs can easily get locked into old habits and modes of thinking that can be difficult to change."

FOOD's IMPACT

Local, free of GMO, additives, chemicals, artificial anything, preservatives, hormones and yucky stuff.......

"I built an awareness of how my relationship with my food was very much my relationship with myself." Sophie Chiche, Creator, *Life By Me*, www.lifebyme.com, featured in *The Inner Weigh*® documentary.

Hippocrates stated "Let thy food be thy medicine and thy medicine be thy food." What you eat, how you eat and when you eat, reflect in your day. If you put junk in, full of additives; artificial colors; hormones; antibiotics; unpronounceable names; you will not only absorb the energy of these into your body, you'll get junk out. In his book, *Food Energetics*, Steve Gagné suggests "Your relationships with certain foods are some of the most intimate relationships in your life. How a food looks, tastes, smells and feels as you eat it, whether it is cold or hot, crunchy or soft-all these physical characteristics of food have tremendous sway over both your feelings for it and how it affects you."

Often, when HHC clients write down what they eat and how it makes them feel, they are amazed. This is something many people do not think about. Most of you know what it feels like to have loved and lost. Yet, you may treat food as an afterthought, taking one of the most important ways of loving and nourishing your physical, spiritual and soul bodies and reducing it to a quick 5 minute adventure of convenient colorful chemicals. When your car requires fuel, you don't absentmindedly insert sugar into the gas tank. I like to say, "Alive, pure and vibrant food is to the soul what love is to the heart: bliss."

The documentary *Hungry for Change* beautifully showcases the disconnect many experience between food, feelings and the consumerism industry. Kris Carr, *Crazy, Sexy, Cancer* filmmaker, mentioned "If it's made in a garden, I eat it. The simpler I get, the healthier I get." Dr. Alejandro Junger, author of *Clean* shared "The problem is we are not eating food anymore; we are eating food like products, made to look better and to have longer shelf life."

Osteopathic physician Dr. Mercola, author and addiction specialist

Jason Vale; David Wolfe, author of *Eating for Beauty,* and I are all proponents of regularly juicing veggies and fruits. In the documentary *Hungry for Change*, Dr. Mercola mentions he juices 20 pounds of veggies every week. Jason Vale reminds you that juice "is easy to absorb and the ultimate fast food."

Invitation to expand:
What if you took time daily, to ask your body what it needs and listened to the first answer that came to you? What type of food does it crave? Does it need rest or physical movement? Does it need water or food? Often, your body craves water yet this craving is confused for food.

I extend an invitation to get to know your food; determine how far it traveled before you placed it in your home and what nutrients are in it. Source local seasonal ingredients, visit farms, ask questions. Befriend a chef or two. Tune in to you, pay attention to your food and you will tune into those around you. As Lima Ohsawa stated "No foods are forgiven except when your body tells you so."

FERMENTED FOOD

Fermented food involves converting sugar (carbohydrates) to alcohol (ethanol). Wine, beer and cider is fermented as is sauerkraut, dry sausages, kimchi, kefir, kombucha, miso, yogurt and vinegar. On her blog, www. cheeseslaves.com, Anne Marie Michaels lists 8 reasons to eat fermented foods. Fermented foods: 1) Improve digestion 2) Restore proper balance of bacteria in the gut (see GAPS section) 3) Are inexpensive 4) Are rich in enzymes 5) Increases vitamin content 6) Help absorb nutrients eaten 7) Last longer because they are preserved 8) Are full of flavor.

For the lactose intolerant, yogurt may still be a viable option. According to Joanne Slavin, a professor in the Department of Food Science and Nutrition at the University of Minnesota, "...Sometimes people who cannot tolerate milk can eat yogurt. This is because the lactose (usually the part people can't tolerate) in milk is broken down as the milk is fermented and turns into yogurt."

Fermented foods are a component of the GAPS protocol (see Gut and

Psychology Syndrome) and in many continents including Europe and Asia.

In her book, *Nourishing Traditions*, nutritionist Sally Fallon discussed the health benefits of ancient foods. Traditionally, fermentation began with washing and cutting vegetables/fruits and mixing with herbs and spices that were briefly pounded and combined with salt water. They were placed in airtight containers at room temperature for several days and stored in a cool, dark place (where they keep for several months). Today culture starters and fermented foods can be purchased, however, many have added vinegar and are pasteurized, destroying beneficial microflora. Historically, American Indians pounded vegetables that were placed in underground vessels and stored for months or years.

In Europe, sauerkraut, cucumbers, beets and turnip are popular fermented foods. The ancient Romans valued sauerkraut for its medicinal properties. In Russia and Poland, green tomatoes, peppers and lettuce were favorite cultured foods.

Terri L. Saunders, in her article entitled *The Magical Power of Fermented Foods,* stated that Asians prepared and ate cultured foods with every meal. The Korean staple, kimchi blends cabbage, carrots, green onions, ginger, garlic and hot peppers. Japan's important fermented foods include shoyu, tamari, miso, rice vinegar, umeboshi plums and mirin. The Chinese government distributes cabbage to the people each fall to ferment and store through winter. Indonesians eat tempeh or fermented soy. Sally states the body can digest only fermented soy foods and that unfermented soy products as soy milk and tofu are harmful to health.

Saunders also mentions that kefir is a fermented dairy product from a region of Turkey where Noah's Ark is said to be discovered. Legend states kefir was a gift from the gods and they told the Turks not to reveal its preparation. However, legend also states the Russians heard of kefir's healing properties and tricked the Turks to obtain the recipe. Today, Russian schoolchildren receive a daily glass of kefir, compliments of the government. Cultured or soured milk products are found in Scandinavia, Middle East and India. Cultured butter and fermented cheeses are also common in Europe.

GINGER

According to www.medicinalherbinfo.org ginger is an ancient herb that produces heat in the body. It is used for spasms, vomiting and nausea and fever, as an analgesic, antiseptic and expectorant. Ginger also causes sweating, is a stimulant and natural blood thinner (anti-coagulant). Also, according to Steve Gagné, ginger stimulates bile and other digestive enzyme production.

During a radio interview with Robert Scott Bell, Dr. Rashid Buttar mentioned using ginger as a blood thinner. He stated the following "Measure it [ginger] against your pinkie, the width and length of your pinkie finger nail and chop it into small pieces. Throw it in a cup and put some hot water in there. Drink that tea and take the remnants of the ginger and eat them. Every other day, you're going to have a very effective, natural anti-coagulant."

GLUTEN

According to Salma Melngailis, author of *Living Raw Foods*, gluten is a protein found in barley, rye, wheat, other grains, seitan (fake meat) and pasta and used as an additive in many foods. Buckwheat, although it sounds like it contains wheat, is free of gluten and full of protein.

People with acute gluten intolerance have Celiac disease. Gluten damages the small intestine lining and thus interferes with nutrient absorption as well as calcium and Vitamin D absorption. Many are unaware of their gluten sensitivities. People with Celiac do not absorb enough nutrients from food and when they eat gluten, feel sick. Also, people with osteoporosis are thought to have Celiac. Tests for gluten sensitivity include: AGA, EMA, and LTG.

HEMP SEEDS

According to www.healingfoods.com, raw hemp seeds "provide a broad spectrum of health benefits, including: weight loss, increased and sustained energy, rapid recovery from disease or injury, lowered cholesterol and blood pressure, reduced inflammation, improvement in circulation and immune system as well as natural blood sugar control."

Salma Melngailis, author of *Living Raw Foods*, states hemp seeds are not seeds but fruits. They contain a high percent of easily digestible protein as well as omega 3 and omega 6 fatty acids, calcium, Gamma Linolenic Acid (GLA), magnesium, potassium and Vitamin A.

Hemp seeds are highly nutritious and taste good, with a flavor similar to pine nuts. They also contain a complete amino acid profile, including all 20 known amino acids and 9 essential amino acids. They can be sprinkled on salads or placed in smoothies and desserts.

KOMBUCHA/MANCHURIAN TEA/TEA KVASS

"100% raw and organic, Kombucha nourishes the body, delights your taste buds, bolsters your immunity and makes your spirits fly. You feel on top of the world. Healthier. Happier. Stronger. It is living food for a living body." GT Dave, founder of www.synergydrinks.com

Kombucha is a fermented beverage/elixir made with sugar, yeast and tea. It is also known as Manchurian Tea, Manchu Fungus, Tea Kvass, Mo-Gu Fungus japonicus and Kwassan. According to www.anahatabalance.com, Kombucha contains Vitamin B1, B2, B6 & B12; amino acids (protein building blocks); many beneficial acids including acetic acid (antiseptic that inhibits bacteria) and glucuronic acid (liver detoxifier).

Dr. Rudolf Sklenar recognized that glucuronic acid in Kombucha removed waste and toxic deposits and developed a recipe that is used today. With kombucha, Dr. Sklenar treated many conditions, including arthritis, constipation and obesity.

MEDICINAL MUSHROOMS

"Mycelium is Earth's natural Internet."
Paul Stamets

Mycologist Paul Stamets, in a 2008 TED talk, stated that mushrooms are beneficial for cleaning polluted soil, making insecticides, treating smallpox and flu. Fungi arrived on the planet 1.3 billion years ago and they grow fast and produce strong antibiotics.

According to *MyCo Herb, Clinical Guide for Practitioners,* medicinal mushrooms, including chaga, cordyceps, maitake, reishi and shiitake are regarded as sacred agents in elevating spirit and gaining divine perspective. Modern research confirmed that they also strengthen immunity and have many properties including antioxidant, antiviral and antibacterial.

Examples of beneficial mushrooms include maitake, reishi, shiitake and chaga. According to *MyCo Herb, Clinical Guide for Practitioners*, benefits of consuming maitake mushrooms including: immune enhancement, help with high blood pressure, high cholesterol and chronic fatigue. Reishi is classified "as an adaptogen, increasing the body's resistance to stresses such as trauma, anxiety and fatigue." It is one of the oldest medicines with a 4,000 year use in Asia.

Information obtained from *MyCo Herb, Clinical Guide for Practitioners* states that reishi mushrooms are also immune enhancing and aid in high blood pressure as well as heart conditions including palpitations and angina. Shiitake mushrooms benefit allergies, yeast infections, arthritis, colds and flu, liver and kidney disease and are considered an anti-aging agent. Beneficial properties of chaga mushrooms include antibacterial, anti-inflammatory and pain relief.

MICROFLORA

Donna Gates, in her book *The Body Ecology* Diet refers to microflora as alchemists and highly intelligent beings that always communicate with your enteric nervous system. Microflora are housed in the intestines and are also known as the second brain. She stated that this second brain controls the primary brain in your head. Scientific research found that the same receptor sites for neuropeptides and other brain chemicals in the brain are also in the gut. This helps explain the "gut feeling" when intuition guides you.

Gates stated that the brain needs nutrients to function. These nutrients include high quality proteins, glucose and essential fats, which come from the intestines. Serotonin and other neurotransmitters are created from these intestinal nutrients and brought to the brain. Microflora produce these substances and help break food down, making it easily digestible.

Gates also states that microflora produce all the essential B vitamins, vitamin K and short-chain fatty acids for nervous and immune system function. Blood is alkalinized when they pull out minerals from food that nourishes cells. This creates an unsuitable environment for harmful bacteria, viruses, yeasts and parasites. Microflora eliminate sugar cravings by eating excess sugars from the diet. If you are deficient in a mineral such as calcium, microflora can change other minerals such as silica, into needed calcium and transform harmful substances (such as toxic byproducts of heavy metals, chemicals and undigested proteins) into useful substances.

MINERALS

According to Hesh Goldstein, MS and host of Hawaii Health Talk, your physical body consists of more than 100 identified elements. Four elements (carbon, hydrogen, nitrogen and oxygen) make up 96% of your body. Elements, called minerals, comprise the remaining 4%. Most minerals are stored in the bones as calcium and phosphorous and in microscopic amounts in the blood and soft tissues. The information below is according to Hesh Goldstein.

CALCIUM

Calcium helps build strong teeth and bones and is needed to maintain overall health and heart health. It works with Vitamin K in blood clotting and helps keep muscle tone healthy and nerves functioning properly. To absorb calcium, magnesium is necessary.

Good sources include: Leafy green vegetables, water, almonds, legumes, dairy products, tofu, blackstrap molasses, alfalfa sprouts.

Calcium deficiency symptoms include: Stunted bone and teeth growth (if deficiency occurs early in life) and stunted growth. Pregnant women, infants and especially growing children need enough calcium. Soft bones in children (rickets) and brittle bones in adults (osteomalacia) may also result.

IODINE

Iodine is necessary for formation of a thyroid hormone that regulates body functions, especially "basal metabolic rate" (minimum energy needed to exist without moving).

Good sources of iodine include: Seaweed, water and vegetables grown near the seashore.

Iodine deficiency symptoms include: thyroid gland enlargement or goiter; weight gain, extremely dry skin and a husky voice and feeling cold in warm weather. Iodine deficiency in pregnancy causes dwarfism and mental retardation.

IRON

Iron is needed to carry oxygen to muscles to release the energy they need to work. It also helps form hemoglobin and prevent anemia.

Good sources of iron include: Leafy green vegetables; dried apricots; prunes; peaches; raisins; dates; legumes; nuts; whole grains; blackstrap molasses; tofu; sesame meal; alfalfa sprouts; peas; pumpkin seeds and nutritional yeast.

Deficiency symptoms include: Weak, tired and lowered resistance to infection. Teenagers and women are prone to iron-deficiency anemia (smaller red blood cells and less oxygen reach the body and muscles).

MAGNESIUM

According to Dr. Batmanghelidj, magnesium is "involved in more than 300 enzymatic reactions with protein, starch and fat metabolism. It is a vital mineral inside cells that gives stability to all energy dependent processes in the brain, heart, kidneys, liver, pancreas, reproductive organs and more."

Magnesium is found in leafy greens, seeds, lentils, broad beans, peas, avocado, almonds, peanuts, brown rice, cocoa beans and barley. In plants, kelp contains the highest level and is also rich in iodine. Magnesium prevents wrinkles, hernias, promotes wound healing, helps promote healthy joints and connective tissue formation. According to Dr. Batmanghelidj, magnesium deficiency is unrecognized and very common and may manifest as high blood pressure and irregular heartbeat.

PHOSPHORUS

Phosphorus is needed for metabolism and energy release from carbohydrates; protein formation and hereditary characteristics passed from one generation to another. It works with calcium in bone formation and teeth structure.

Good sources of phosphorus include: Legumes, whole grains, dairy products, nuts, tofu, nutritional yeast, bran, lima beans, peas, pumpkin seeds, blackstrap molasses, sesame seed and almond meal.

Deficiency symptoms include: Bone softness or brittleness. Phosphorus intake may be too high instead of too low, especially in meat eaters and processed food eater's diets.

SODIUM and POTASSIUM

Sodium and potassium maintain a balance inside and outside body cells for proper nerve and muscle cell function and help balance the acid/alkaline system. Sodium is needed for the body to absorb various nutrients. Potassium is needed to release energy from proteins, fats and carbohydrates. Both regulate the body's water balance.

Sources of sodium: water, dairy products, miso and olives.

Sodium deficiency symptoms include: Excessive salt intake may result in high blood pressure, hypertension and stroke. However, with excessive sweating or fever, sodium and body fluids may be depleted, causing muscle cramps.

Good sources of potassium: Leafy green vegetables; tomatoes; potatoes; dates; cantaloupe; bananas; apricots; citrus fruits; peas; bamboo shoots; prunes; butternut squash; legumes; papaya; avocado; brussel sprouts; beet greens; blackstrap molasses and alfalfa sprouts.

Potassium deficiency is characterized by muscular weakness, heart muscle irregularities; respiratory and kidney failures. Medicinal diuretic use may also cause potassium loss.

ZINC

According to Dr. Batmanghelidj, zinc is needed for accurate gene expression in DNA assembly and "is involved in the manufacture of more than 200 different enzymes and proteins in all cells of the body." The protein for the insulin receptor on cell membranes also needs a lot of zinc.

Sources of zinc are seeds such as sesame and pumpkin, beef, cheese, pecans, peanuts, lima beans and peas.

Contributors to zinc deficiency include alcohol, low stomach acid; too much calcium, iron and fiber; too little protein and liver and pancreatic disease.

TRACE MINERALS

Trace minerals include chromium, copper, zinc, manganese and sulfur found in whole grains, legumes, nuts, dairy products, leafy greens, fresh and dried fruit and raw and cooked vegetables.

Deficiencies or imbalances may occur from refining grain, which removes some iron, manganese, chromium, zinc and essential minerals from the food supply. Also, since minerals are absorbed from the soil, modern agricultural methods may affect the supply of iodine, copper, zinc and chromium in produce.

NUTRITION

"Nutrition is a strong determining factor in the ability of a human being to make new neural pathways. The human brain is a delicate organ. It requires a precise mixture of water; blood sugar; temperature; electrolyte minerals; essential fatty acids and other nutrients to function correctly."
Mike Adams, Health Ranger, founder of www.naturalnews.com

According to Institute for Integrative Nutrition's (IIN) founder/director, Joshua Rosenthal, 'no one diet fits all'. IIN is the only school in the world integrating every dietary theory, from traditional Eastern philosophies like Chinese medicine and macrobiotics to the modern concepts like glycemic index, raw foods and the Zone. It includes nutrition concepts such as blood type, food energetics, seasonal eating, minerals and the food/mood connection. Modern health issues like adrenal health, inflammation and holistic dentistry are also addressed. IIN was life changing for me and may also be for you.

IIN taught me the importance of primary food- a concept of   nourishment from thoughts, relationships, spirituality and physical activity in addition to food nutrients. As I learned in Chinese medicine, everything is interrelated and disease results from an imbalance of more than one system. Nutrition is of the mind, body and soul. It encompasses more than the food one eats, more than the thoughts one thinks and more than the actions one takes. For more information, visit www.pagona.com and www.instituteforintegrativenutrition.com.

PHYTIC ACID

According to March 26, 2010 article on www. westonaprice.org, entitled *Preparing Grains, Nuts, Seeds and Beans for Maximum Nutrition*, phytic acid in grains, nuts, seeds and beans is a serious problem.

The article states that phytic acid is found in many plant tissues (especially the bran part of grains and seeds) and contains tightly bound phosphorus not readily bioavailable. Phytic acid molecule "arms" bind with minerals including calcium, magnesium, iron and zinc, making them unavailable in the body.

Phytic acid grabs on to (chelates) important minerals and inhibits food digesting enzymes. These enzymes include pepsin (breaks down protein in stomach), amylase (breaks down starch into sugar) and trypsin (needed for protein digestion in small intestine).

Phytic acid is found in commonly consumed foods including brown rice, beans and nuts. To remove the phytic acid from brown rice, soak it in water for 24 hours before rinsing and cooking. To decrease the amount of phytic acid from seeds and nuts, toast them before eating.

PROTEIN

Proteins are essential as building blocks for your body. According to Dr.

Batmanghelidj, without proteins, enzymes, receptors and neurotransmitters could not be made. He suggests (because proteins tend to make the body acidic) eating a good balance of fruits and vegetables and protein. Good non-meat protein sources are legumes such as fava, lentils, mung beans, chickpeas and green beans, green vegetables like spinach, tofu, hemps seeds and chia seeds. Fresh meat, eggs, fish, cheese also contain protein.

According to John Douillard, D.O. severe protein deficiency may manifest as one or more of the following symptoms:

1) edema 2) nausea 3) fainting 4) headache 5) depression/anxiety 6) sleep issues 7) skin ulcers 8) slow healing 9) weak and tired 10) skin rash/dry skin 11) thinning brittle hair/hair loss 12) ridges in fingers/toe nails 13) muscle soreness and cramps 14) crave carbs and candy or is someone who is snacker.

RAW FOOD

"I wake up feeling clear and energized in the morning. What is most profound for me about this light eating pattern is the flow of cosmic energy I feel coursing through my body. During the day it feels as if joy is running through every cell independent of external factors."
Gabriel Cousens, M.D. (raw food doctor), author of *Conscious Eating*

In the *Hungry For Change* documentary, health journalist Mike Adams, mentioned that parsley and cilantro are effective at detoxing the body because parsley cleanses the blood supply and cilantro binds heavy metals like mercury and removes them from your system. In an article entitled *Raw Fresh Produce vs. Cooked Food*, Arthur M. Baker, MA, MHE stated that cooking denatures protein (decreases/destroys biological activity); coagulates protein (visualize frying an egg when the clear protein gel thickens into glue like consistency); degrades protein, amino acids and carbohydrates (an example is dark crust on bread, which occurs during baking in the Maillard reaction). Baker also stated that cooking destroys vitamins, minerals and enzymes (when food is heated more than 117° F). He stated that "When the pH of a baked item rises above 6, nearly all of the thiamin is destroyed."

Enzymes help digest food. When food is heated more than 117 °F, enzymes become inactive. The body uses energy to generate more of its own digestive enzymes. Food cooked in lower temperature (less than 117 °F) is not denatured. Using dehydrators (set less than 117 °F) to blow hot air on food, allow you to make creative recipes including uncooked dehydrated garbanzo beans for falafel and dehydrated raw crackers.

Registered dietitian Roxanne Moore, spokeswoman for the American Dietetic Association, stated the less cooked the fruit or vegetable, the more nutrients and fiber it retains. If you don't like raw vegetables, how they are cooked determines the amount of nutrients that survive. A few tips: use fresh produce and shorter cooking times and steam instead of boil.

RECIPES

All recipes are free of gluten & processed stuff....

CHILLED AVOCADO CITRUS SOUP
(learned from Elephant Walk's Executive Chef Nadsa De Monteiro, www.elephantwalk.com)

This is an easy & healthy favorite cold soup.

Serves 4
2 TBS extra virgin olive oil or coconut oil
½ TSP black pepper
1 quart freshly squeezed orange juice
1 TSP garlic (chopped)
1 C freshly squeezed lime juice
1 sm. onion (chopped)
1 TBS unrefined, unprocessed sugar
1 TBS Sea salt
2/3 C button mushrooms (sliced ¼ inch thick)
3 avocados (cut in ½ inch cubes)
2 C plum tomatoes (diced without pulp)
1 TBS cilantro, chopped (per serving)

PAGONA

1. Cover the chopped onion with salt for 20-30 min.
2. Rinse the salt off the onion, drain & squeeze off excess water.
3. Mix salt, pepper, orange juice, lime juice, garlic & sugar well.
4. Add olive oil & mix well.
5. Add diced avocado, mushroom, tomatoes and onion & stir gently to mix well.
6. Allow to chill 1 hour before serving.

'ANTS' ON A LOG
(from *Integrative Nutrition* by Joshua Rosenthal)
A simple, high protein kid friendly snack.

Prep Time: 10 min
Serves 1

2 TBS almond butter or preferred nut butter
2 stalks organic celery
Handful dried blueberries or preferred dried fruit (free of additives like sugar and preservatives)
Wash celery. Spread nut butter inside each stalk. Dot with blueberries.

BERRY MANGO HEMP SHAKE
(adapted from recipe in *Living Raw Food* by Sarma Melngailis)

A favorite go to shake, I drink variations of this regularly.
Prep time: 5 min   Yield: 4 ½ cups

1 C hemp seeds
3 C filtered water
1 TBS coconut oil (unrefined, hexane free)
3 TBS honey
8 oz. fresh or frozen strawberries
8 oz. mango

-Puree all in high speed blender until smooth.

Have fun: Experiment with your favorite fruit- fresh or frozen, vanilla bean & cacao nibs & enjoy endless possibilities.

CHOCOLATE COCONUT TRUFFLES
(courtesy of *Living Raw Food* by Sarma Melngailis)

Makes about 40 truffles

I made these for the Holidays & fell in love with them. A neighbor & fellow chocolate connoisseur remarked they taste fresh & delicious! They are also easy to prepare & without additives like soy lecithin.

½ C coconut oil, warmed to liquefy
¼ tsp sea salt
1 C dried shredded coconut (unsweetened)
2 tsp vanilla extract
2 ½ C cocoa powder, sifted
¼ C agave nectar

1. In high speed blender, blend coconut oil, agave, vanilla & salt.
2. Add shredded coconut, ½ C at a time & blend until smooth.
3. Transfer mix to bowl & stir in 2 C of cocoa powder until it's mixed well.
4. Place bowl in fridge for 10 min or more to slightly set.
5. Place remaining ¼ C cocoa powder in small plate.
6. Spoon heaping teaspoons of chocolate mixture & roll them into balls. Roll these in the cocoa powder.
7. Store truffles in fridge.

PAGONA

COUGH SYRUP
(courtesy of *Vital Foods for Total Health* by Bernard Jensen, D.C.)

It may sound weird, yet it is a simple & natural way to soothe coughs.

6 onions (cut up)
½ C pure organic honey

1) Place onions in a double boiler with the honey.
2) Cook on low heat for 2 hours and strain.
3) Take slightly warm (as needed).

PICKLED CUCUMBERS
(taken from *Introducing Macrobiotic Cooking* by Wendy Esko)

2-3 lbs. cucumbers
1 large onion (halved then quartered)
10-12 C water
1-2 sprigs of fresh or dry dill
¼-1/3 C sea salt

1. Combine water & salt. Bring to a boil & simmer 3 min until salt dissolves. Allow to cool.
2. Place cucumbers, dill & onion slices in large jar. Pour cooled salt water over them & let sit in a dark, cool place for 3-4 days.
3. Cover & refrigerate. They will keep for about 1 month in fridge.

LEMONADE
(adapted from www.eatingwell.com recipe)

As a lemonade lover, I love healthier versions of this refresher)

Prep time: 20 min
1 cucumber (sliced)
½ C cold filtered water
1/3 C mild honey
3 C ice
½ C fresh lime juice
¼ tsp sea salt

-Combine all ingredients in a high speed blender & enjoy!
Have fun: Add mint, lemon or desired garnish into lemonade or on top.

PAGONA's LENTIL SOUP
(vegetarian, 'smoky', Indian style)

I use recipes only when I bake. Growing up with mom's lentil soup was great inspiration for this version. The digestive enzymes in the miso add another health benefit.

16 oz. (1lb) lentils
1 tsp ground black pepper
8 C filtered water
1 onion (diced)
5 TBS coconut oil
1 tsp mustard powder
1 tsp all-purpose seasoning
2 whole bay leaves
*2 TBS miso paste (organic, unpasteurized)
1 C tomato sauce
1 tsp Kala Namak (Indian black sea salt)
1/8 tsp cinnamon

PAGONA

1. Rinse lentils. Bring 8 C of water to a boil.
2. Add lentils & stir remaining ingredients (except miso) in pot.
3. Cook on medium heat for 15-20 min or until lentils are soft & firm.
4. *Turn off heat. Mix 2 TBS miso with broth & add to pot. (I love South River Miso for organic, unpasteurized & Japanese traditional miso). View how miso is prepared at www.southrivermiso.com.

KITCHARI
(courtesy of *Integrative Nutrition* by Joshua Rosenthal)

Rice & mung beans used in Ayurvedic medicine to clean the system.

Bean soak time: 2 hrs.   Prep: 10 min   Cooking Time: 1 hr.   Serves 6

1 C basmati rice
4 C water
½ C mung beans
½ tsp sea salt
2 TBS ghee or olive oil
½ tsp turmeric powder
1tsp mustard seeds
1 tsp cumin seeds

1. Soak beans in a bowl with water for 2 hrs. drain & rinse.
2. Cook beans in 4 C water for 30 min, drain excess liquid.
3. Heat ghee or olive oil over medium heat in deep pan.
4. Add mustard & cumin seeds & stir fry until they pop, about 2 min.
5. Add rice, beans, turmeric & salt & stir. Add water & bring to boil.
6. Reduce heat, cover most of way & simmer 25 min until cooked.
Optional: add veggies while rice & beans are cooking.

SOUL INGREDIENTS

CASHEW MAYO
(from *Recipes for Longer Life* by Dr. Ann Wigmore)

This is a tasty mayo alternative without dairy.

Makes 4 cups

1 C water
½ C raw cashews
½ tsp paprika
1 C coconut oil
1 tsp kelp
2 lemons, juiced

1. Blend cashews, water, kelp & paprika.
2. Slowly, add lemon & oil.

CLASSIC PAD THAI
(courtesy of *Hot Sour Salty Sweet* written by
Jeffrey Alford and Naomi Duguid)

An authentic version of the classic. When I prepare it, people continuously ask what restaurant it came from.

*Note: wok is needed. Serves 3-4 as a meal. Cooking time 6 min.

2 oz. boneless free range, organic pork (chicken or beef) 1 ½ inch thin, long slices. Substitute vegetables if you prefer & omit fish sauce.
1 tsp unbleached sugar
1 TBS soy sauce
1 TBS fish sauce
3 large free range eggs
Pinch salt

PAGONA

3 TBS coconut oil
2-3 garlic cloves (minced)
1 TBS dried shrimp
½ lb. narrow dried rice noodles (soak 20 min in warm H2O & drain)
1 heaping tsp tamarind pulp (dissolved in 2-3 TBS warm H2O) or
substitute 1 TBS rice vinegar + 1 TBS H2O
1 C dry roasted peanuts (chop coarsely)
½ lb. (4 C) bean sprouts rinsed & drained
3 scallions, trimmed & smashed flat with cleaver & cut 1 ½ inch

Accompaniments/condiments:
1 C chile vinegar sauce   unbleached sugar   Cayenne pepper
½- 1 European cuke (thinly sliced)   1 lime (sm wedges)

1. Add sugar to pork & toss.
2. In separate bowl, mix tamarind or rice vinegar w H2O, soy sauce & fish sauce.
3. In another sm. bowl, beat eggs lightly with salt.
4. Heat wok over high heat & add ½ TBS oil.
5. When hot, stir fry garlic until changes color (about 15 sec).
6. Add pork & fry until changes color (1 min or less).
7. Pour in eggs & cook until they set around pork (< 1 min).
8. Use spatula to cut into large pieces & transfer to plate & set aside.
9. Place wok back on high heat & add 1 ½ TBS oil, swirl to coat.
10. Toss noodles & stir fry quickly, pressing vs. hot wok to sear. Heat & turn & press again.
11. Move noodles to side of wok & toss 2C bean sprouts & scallions.
12. Stir fry quickly 20 sec pressing vs. wok.
13. Add dried shrimp & toss briefly with spatula.
14. Add soy sauce mix & stir fry 30 sec.
15. Add egg & mix together. Add desired accompaniments.
Marinate at least 30 min before serving.

SEAWEED SALAD
(from *Integrative Nutrition* by Joshua Rosenthal)
(I love seaweed- especially when it is fresh & nicely seasoned).

Prep Time: 5 min
Marinade Time: 30 min
Serves 4

¾ oz. 3 varieties seaweed combined
1 tsp honey
2 TBS brown rice vinegar
1 tsp sesame oil
1 tsp sesame seeds

SEA VEGETABLES/ALGAE

Joshua Rosenthal, in his book, *Integrative Nutrition,* mentioned 6 types of sea vegetables (marine algae): arame, dulse, hijiki, kombu, nori, wakame. Another type, kelp, refers to the brown seaweeds including wakame, kombu and alaria. Other marine algae include Irish moss, red laver (nori), sea palm and dulse. Freshwater algae include chlorella and spirulina.

Sea vegetables are superfoods, containing vitamins and concentrated minerals. They aid in: improving digestion; strengthening teeth and bones and reducing blood cholesterol. They can be found in Asian markets and local health food stores. Look for those grown wild and harvested locally.

In his book, *Food Energetics: The Spiritual, Emotional and Nutritional Power of What We Eat*, Steve Gagné stated that algae are one of the most ancient plants on earth and "Once ingested, algae begin to work like a janitor, cleaning, purifying and strengthening the internal environment." He also mentioned that regular use of algae aids in bringing deep emotional and psychological issues to the surface, helping face them. As in any release of toxins, adjustment symptoms may occur including headaches, nausea and not feeling well.

SUGAR

**"Sugar is without question the cocaine of the food world but
they get away with hiding that drug within "food."**
From documentary *Hungry For Change*

Mike Lambert, acupuncturist, psychologist and former Health and Safety investigator stated, "A single lump of refined sugar would kill you if the body didn't begin a survival response to cope with it." As refined sugar is acidic, the body protects itself by releasing large amounts of calcium (from bones and teeth) into the system. The pineal gland in the brain is affected as is the production of serotonin, a neurotransmitter. Serotonin depletion triggers depression. Think of the people you know who are depressed. How many crave sweets like chocolate, high energy drinks or soda? Did you know a can of soda has 9 teaspoons of sugar? Did you know alcohol addiction=sugar addiction?

A hormone called insulin carries sugar (in the form of glucose) to the cells. Too much sugar causes either: the underproduction of insulin by the pancreas or too much insulin. In either case, glucose is not being absorbed and is stored as fat. Insulin imbalance may lead to diabetes, metabolic syndrome and other issues such as thyroid imbalance. The thyroid or 'master gland' regulates metabolism, body temperature and hormones. Therefore, an imbalanced, depleted immune system does not promote health and other diseases may result. As David Icke stated, "The body is a hologram and every part of a hologram is a smaller version of the whole. This includes the mind and emotions." This interrelatedness is everywhere including the Universe, physical body, spiritual world and soul body.

Many clients are surprised to hear about sugar's toxic effects and are unaware of sugar addiction (it is an addiction like alcohol and drugs). My journey with sugar was that of addiction until I took responsibility and became aware, informed and took action. Dr. Chopra, in his book, *The Path to Love* stated "When love is replaced by an object, the result is addiction." Many people forget the importance of a life full of love and balance. Your body tells you when it needs something; you must bring awareness and understanding to it and act.

As I began researching, studying and understanding Eastern and Western philosophies about health, spirituality, etc., I had an epiphany. Sugar, toxicity, negativity and all imbalances (whether on a physical level or energetic level, conscious or unconscious) in my life, contributed to many of the problems/issues in my life. How liberated I am to be free of them on all levels and help others understand the psychological, physical and spiritual roots of illness, stress and imbalance. Sugar may be one factor yet it is a pervasive one.

Tips to decrease sugar:
1. Eliminate all refined, bleached sugar from the home.
2. Replace it with organic fruit, raw organic honey, date sugar and rapadura.
3. Make snacks with cocoa, unrefined coconut oil, honey, ground hemp seeds, ground chia seeds and nuts and store in freezer. Experiment with flavors!
4. Eat sweet vegetables like watermelon radish and sweet potato.

TEA

According to *The Story of Tea*, by Mary Lou and Robert Heiss, tea is served worldwide and enjoyed by millions. Tea originated in China and spread to the rest of Asia and to the West.

Why is tea good for you? According to Adeline Yen Mah, author of *Watching the Tree,* her Aunt Baba told Adeline when she was a child that "tea sharpens the mind, soothes the stomach and nourishes your qi." Based on information in *The Story of Tea*, tea contains the amino acid theanine (helps one relax); antioxidants; minerals; flavonoids (higher in green tea); proteins; polysaccharides; polyphenols (stop oxidation); vitamins B1, B2 and C. Researchers suggest that green tea may help lower cholesterol, blood pressure and aid in weight loss.

Aung San Suu Kyi described the Japanese tea ceremony and its relationship to her purpose and wisdom. She stated, "The tea ceremony, illustrated the necessity of removing all the ugly or disharmonious before reaching out to beauty...to acquire good taste one has to be able to recognize both ugliness and beauty is applicable to the whole range of human experience."

As the daughter of General Aung San, "the father of Burma's independence" and Burma's greatest hero, Suu Kyi continued his fight for Burma's independence. She was the recipient of the 1991 Nobel Peace Prize yet was unable to receive it as she was under house arrest.

TOXICITIES

During his talk 29 April 2009, entitled *Impact on Chronic Disease and Premature Aging* (www.factsontoxicity.com), Rashid A. Buttar, D.O., Board certified in Clinical Metal Toxicology and Preventive Medicine addressed disease contributing factors. He stated that free radical damage occurs in our bodies when atoms lose their neutrality (now net positive charged) and look to stabilize by adding negative electrons from surrounding atoms. An example of oxidation or free radical damage is a sliced apple turning brown. Another example is heart disease. Antioxidants are needed to counter the free radicals. The body makes antioxidants yet is unable to when 7 toxicities occur, resulting in disease. According to Dr. Buttar, the following are the 7 toxicities:

1. **Heavy metals** [mercury (2nd most toxic after plutonium) in amalgams and vaccines and inhalation of mercury vapor and heavy metals in water supply]. Other heavy metals include lead, plutonium and cadmium.
2. **POP's** (Persistent Organic Pollutants) include insecticides. He refers to POP's as persistent because the body is unable to dispose of them. He mentioned that insecticides used in 1950's (no longer used) resulted in birth defects three generations later.
3. **'Opportunistics'** (Bacteria, viruses, parasites, etc.). These have an opportunity to "set up house" via heavy metals or POP's. He stated, as we also know in Chinese medicine, that if the symptom is only treated, the root cause exists and disease manifestation reoccurs.
4. **Energetics** (electromagnetic high power, cell phones, TV, microwaves, etc.).

5. **Emotional Psychological Issues.** These may be recent or unresolved from childhood. Most are self- created and deeply ingrained. He believes "this is the worst form of oxidative stress."
6. **Food Toxicity**, specifically- Immunological and Irradiation Issues and Genetic Engineering of Food (GM/GMO). He posed the question if DNA in food is manipulated, what affect does it have on human DNA?
7. **Spiritual Toxicity.** Dr. Buttar stated "There have been more people killed in the name of God than any other cause of death in the history of man. Understanding that "religion" is the source of the 7th toxicity is the 1st step in resolving the 7th toxicity."

Dr. Buttar, FAAPM, FACAM, FAAIM, founded the Centers for Advanced Healing and trains physicians in their protocol. The Centers for Advanced Healing specialize in chronic and difficult to diagnose conditions; neurodegenerative diseases; metabolic disorders and heavy metal and chemical toxicity. For more information, visit www.factsontoxicology.com and www.centersforadvancedhealing.com

UMEBOSHI PLUMS

According to www.mitoku.com, umeboshi plums stimulate digestion, eliminate toxins and decrease fatigue. They are regarded as a hangover remedy and when taken daily, are one of the best preventive medicines.

Umeboshi plum extract is used in Asian folk treatments to alkalize acidic blood and stomach conditions. Almost 200 years ago, the Japanese experimented with ways to concentrate umeboshi's healing powers. A dark liquid called bainiku ekisu (plum extract) was developed. To make the extract, sour green ume plums are slowly cooked to obtain their most active highly concentrated form. The resulting dark, sticky, thick liquid is mixed with hot water and honey and drunk as a tonic. Dried plum extract is also formed into pills, called meitan. In plum extract and meitan, the plums' citric acid content is concentrated tenfold, equivalent to about twenty-five times the content in lemon juice.

Like many of Japan's ancient medicinal foods, the pickled plum's origin is unclear. One theory traces it to China, where a dried smoked plum, or ubai, was discovered in a tomb over two thousand years ago. The ubai is one of China's oldest medicines used to counteract nausea, reduce fevers and coughs.

The oldest Japanese record of pickled plums used as medicine is in a medical text written about one thousand years ago. Umeboshi were used to prevent fatigue, purify water, rid toxins in the body and cure diseases such as dysentery, typhoid and food poisoning.

VITAMINS

Vitamins are vital to our health. Below, Hesh Goldstein who holds a Masters in Nutrition and host of Health Talk, (www.healthtalkhawaii.com) discussed the most important vitamins. This list is taken from an article found on wwwnaturalnews.com.

BIOTIN
Biotin keeps connective tissues healthy and strong and supports healthy hair, skin and nails.

FOLATE (FOLIC ACID)
Folic acid may help decrease neuro tube defects. Mothers and those wishing to conceive need adequate amounts. Folic acid helps form red blood cells, improve circulation and digest protein.

VITAMIN A
Vitamin A is a carotenoid antioxidant critical for healthy eyes, skin and the liver. It is also important for skeletal system growth and health.

VITAMIN B1 (Thiamine)
Vitamin B1 helps your body convert starches and sugar into energy. It supports a healthy heart, promotes digestion and helps prevent fatigue.

VITAMIN B2 (Riboflavin)
Vitamin B2 helps your body release energy to cells and use protein, fats and sugars.

VITAMIN B3 (Niacin)
Vitamin B3 helps maintain healthy nerves and skin and healthy cholesterol levels.

VITAMIN B6
Vitamin B6 supports nervous system health, aids protein, carbohydrate and fat metabolism and controls cholesterol level. It also helps the chemical balance between blood and tissue, prevents water retention and builds hemoglobin.

VITAMIN B12
Vitamin B12 is essential for adrenal health and helps convert food into energy. Often, low energy can be treated by increasing vitamin B12 in your diet.

VITAMIN C
As an antioxidant, Vitamin C fights free radicals, provides immune support, prevents scurvy and helps support healthy skin. Vitamin C is needed to make collagen.

VITAMIN D
In the book, *Put Your Heart in Your Mouth,* Dr. Natasha Campbell-McBride discussed natural treatment for high blood pressure, heart attack, stroke and atherosclerosis. She mentioned many vitamin deficiencies including Vitamin D deficiency. Dr. Natasha stated, "Vitamin D is made from cholesterol in our skin when it is exposed to sunlight."

Vitamin D deficiency includes: diabetes; heart disease; mental illness; obesity; auto immune illness (lupus, rheumatoid arthritis and others); osteoarthritis; cancer; chronic pain; hyperparathyroidism (manifests as kidney stones; aches; chronic fatigue; depression; digestive abnormalities and muscle weakness).

How do you nourish yourself with Vitamin D? Vitamin D works with Vitamin A. Sunlight and cholesterol rich foods like cod liver oil, fish, butter and egg yolks provide Vitamin D. Dr. Natasha stated that although Vitamin B2 supplements are available, this vitamin is not as effective and not the same as natural Vitamin D and toxicity may result.

VITAMIN E

According to information obtained from http://www.umm.edu/altmed/ articles/vitamin-e-000341.htm#ixzz1yl14sLEe, Vitamin E is fat-soluble and an antioxidant found in many foods, fats and oils. It also helps make red blood cells and use vitamin K.

People who have trouble absorbing fat may develop Vitamin E deficiency. Symptoms of serious vitamin E deficiency include: abnormal eye movements, muscle weakness, loss of muscle mass, vision problems and unsteady walking. A long lasting deficiency may cause liver and kidney problems.

VITAMIN K

According to information from: http://www.umm.edu/altmed/articles/ vitamin-k-000343.htm#ixzz1yl306koJ, Vitamin K is a fat soluble vitamin needed for blood clotting and bone health. It is rare to have a vitamin K deficiency because in addition to being in leafy green foods, intestinal bacteria can make vitamin K. Sometimes taking antibiotics kills this bacteria and leads to a mild deficiency, especially in those with low levels.

Vitamin K deficiency can lead to excessive bleeding, which may begin oozing from gums or nose. Other things that may lead to vitamin K deficiency include: health problems that prevent Vitamin K absorption, such as gallbladder or biliary disease; cystic fibrosis; Celiac and Crohn's disease; liver disease; taking blood-thinners, such as Coumadin; long-term hemodialysis and serious burns.

WATER

"Nothing in the world is softer and weaker than water; but for attacking the hard and the strong, there is nothing like it. For nothing can take its place. That the weak overcomes the strong and the soft overcomes the hard. This is something known by all but practiced by none."
Ch. 78 of *Tao Te Ching* translated by John C.H. Wu

SOUL INGREDIENTS

In the book, *Obesity, Cancer and Depression,* F. Batmanghelidj, M.D., states that water: 1) is "the main source of energy- "cash flow" of the body." 2) forms a membrane (protective barrier) around the cell. 3) water is necessary for the neurotransmission systems –i.e. water generates energy allowing potassium into the cell and pushing sodium outside. 4) is "the central regulator of energy and osmotic balance in the body." 5) is the "vehicle of transport for circulating blood cells- the core of the immune system." 6) breaks down and energizes food and increases the rate of essential substances in food. 7) is needed for neurotransmitter and hormone production and prevents memory loss, fatigue and stress.

Dr. Batmanghelidj spent two years and 7 months in Evin Prison as a political prisoner in 1979 at the onset of the Iranian Revolution. He gave a prisoner with peptic ulcer pain 2 glasses of water and the prisoner was pain free in 8 minutes. He treated 3,000 prisoners with peptic ulcer disease with only water. In *Obesity, Cancer and Depression,* he spoke about dehydration (concentrated acidic blood) contributing to toxic deposits in the joints, kidneys, liver, brain, skin, fat stores and tissue spaces as well as pain; depression; obesity and degenerative conditions including arthritis and MS. Dr. Batmanghelidj also stated that "You need to prevent thirst to lose weight and you must make sure you do not become deficient in minerals."

How much water is enough? Dr. Batmanghelidj mentioned the body needs "No less than 2 quarts of water and some salt every day to compensate for its natural losses in urine, respiration and perspiration." For an average sized person, he recommends 4 quarts/day. As a general rule for heavier people, he suggests drinking ½ oz. of water daily for every pound of body weight. For example, a 200 lb. person would drink 100 oz. of water. Also, it is vital for everyone to drink at least 2 glasses of water upon waking.

In *The Secret Life of Water,* Masaru Emoto displayed his research photographing water when it freezes and discovered water is influenced by toxins and what it hears. Emoto teaches that water is life, beauty, a mirror and prayer. He stated "About 70% of our bodies are water. Just like water, people must always be allowed to flow freely." He displayed photos of water crystals when loving and not so loving thoughts were conveyed to them. Emoto reported that "Love and thankfulness show the most beautiful crystals in the world."

In her book *Energy Secrets,* Alla Svirinskaya presented many energy techniques to improve health. One technique she mentioned involves an energy shower. She suggests preparing a thick salt rub paste by adding a bit of sweet almond oil and 2-3 drops of sage or juniper essential oil to a handful of sea salt. (Avoid sage if pregnant). While standing in the shower, rub paste all over your body (avoiding head and face if you choose). Next, shower, with water running over your head, while confidently and sincerely requesting the water wash away all negative energy. Following the shower, remain in bare feet while you dress in comfortable clothes wearing no jewelry, not even a watch.

WHEATGRASS

According to Golda Sirota, author of *Love Food,* fresh wheatgrass is a superfood rich in chlorophyll, heals anemia and protects from carbon monoxide, gas and radiation exposure. It also helps release toxins.

Ann Wigmore introduced wheatgrass to America in 1955. In her book, *The Wheatgrass Book,* she mentioned that wheatgrass stimulates the thyroid gland, detoxifies the liver and protects the blood. Ann suggests drinking it in small amounts throughout the day, on an empty or close to empty stomach. She also promoted many benefits of chlorophyll including: rich in oxygen (helps with food oxidation and clearer thinking); rich in protein; improves blood sugar imbalances; high magnesium content helps restore fertility; increases energy; brings color back into gray and if grown in organic soil, absorbs 92 of the known 102 minerals from the soil.

SOUL INGREDIENTS

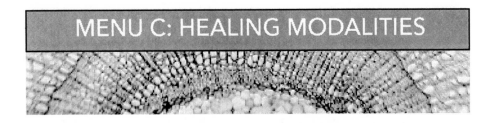

MENU C: HEALING MODALITIES

ESOTERIC INGREDIENTS & other ingredients

AKASHIC RECORDS

These records were not consciously in my life until I began studying with Sue and Aaron Singleton, owners of The Way to Balance. During my first session, over 10 years ago, Sue remarked it may take time before I allow and open up. Much to her surprise and mine, my soul and body were ready. During my second healing session, abundant tears flew down my cheeks paving the way for continued cleansing and clearing. Over the years, Sue's repeated requests to look inward instead of outward fueled confusion in me. How would I do that I asked myself? That concept, although very loved and respected in my daily life was a fearful and unwelcomed guest then. It sat far removed from anything I considered friendly. It was my thinking that made it so. Sue taught many things including the concept of Akashic records.

According to Linda Howe, The Akashic Records are "a soul level spiritual resource out of which all things are formed." The Records are known in all spiritual traditions and exist everywhere as an invisible, vibrational library of all knowledge of each person's soul journey, including the cosmos. Everyone can access their records and receive Divine guidance. The Akashic Records exist in a quantum state and are in the DNA.

Dr. Zhi Gang Sha, in *The Power of Soul* stated there is a book in the Akashic Records for each person's soul. This book, he shared, records all your activities, service, behaviors and thoughts in this and previous lifetimes.

ANIMALS

Animals, like children, remind you of the importance of unconditional love. They also work together, reconcile after arguments and care about the wellbeing of others within their group. Unlike humans, sea animals have capabilities including bioluminescence and camouflage.

Frans de Waal studied morality in animals. Morality is based on reciprocity, empathy and compassion. De Waal studied how animals fight, reconcile, share and cooperate. During a Ted Peachtree talk in November 2011 entitled Moral behavior in animals, he stated that after a fight, chimpanzees reconcile. Bonobos also reconcile. When conflict damages a valuable relationship, they sense that something must be done.

Frans de Waal shared that in chimps there is a "Full understanding of the need of cooperation and willingness to work." They understand favors will be returned. Elephants studied in Thailand were found to have empathy, like humans.

Yawn contagion is also something we share with animals. Frans de Waal stated this is "related to the body channel of synchronization that underlies empathy" and is universal in mammals. Two Kampuchea monkeys had a task to complete. When it was completed, one received cucumber and the other grapes. (This created inequity). The monkey that received cucumber ate the first cucumber and refused the rest. This experiment was done with dogs, birds and chimpanzees with similar findings.

Dr. Susan Savage-Rumbaugh's lifelong work with bonobo apes and chimps is fascinating. In her Tedtalk entitled The real-life culture of bonobos, she spoke about bonobos (in Congo) that are empathetic and egalitarian and use sexual behavior for communication and conflict resolution. Bonobos understand spoken language and learn tasks by watching. She showed a video where bonobos walk upright, play the xylophone and Pac Man and drive a go cart. It is wonderful to watch and demonstrates how culture determines much of what a species does.

David Gallo, in his March 2007 Tedtalk, spoke about the underwater accomplishments of sea animals. He shared that bioluminescence helps avoid being eaten and attracts prey. Only 3% of the underwater world has been explored. Gallo showed many underwater animals including an octopus that camouflages by matching the pattern, color, brightness and texture of algae.

APPLIED KINESIOLOGY

What is kinesiology? Kinesiology is the study of movement. In the U.S, this includes: exercise and sport biomechanics; history; philosophy; physiology; biochemistry and molecular/cellular physiology; psychology; sociology; motor behavior; measurement; physical fitness and sports medicine.

George Goodheart developed Applied Kinesiology (AK) therapy using muscle testing. Using an integrated approach involving a triad of health (chemical, mental and structural factors) AK, through an invisible link to higher intelligence, allows you to know if something (object, idea, thought or person) is good or bad for you.

According to www.appliedkinesiology.com, AK therapies include joint mobilization; myofascial therapies; cranial techniques; meridian therapy; clinical nutrition; dietary management and reflex procedures. Often, tests for environmental or food sensitivities are done using a previously strong muscle to find what weakens it.

AK can be explained by an equilateral triangle with structural health at the base and chemical and mental health on each side. When a person has poor health, he/she has an imbalance in one or more of three factors. A health problem on one side can affect the other sides. For example, a chemical imbalance may cause mental symptoms.

ART

"Art is not supposed to change the world, to change practical things, but to change perceptions. Art can change the way we see the world. Art can create an analogy."

JR Alain Arias-Misson stated "The purpose of art is not rarified, intellectual distillate-it is life, intensified, brilliant life." Art is a reflection of life and echoes our emotions, lifestyles and dreams. It is interpreted with the eyes and history of each observer recognizing that each interpretation is correct. Alex Grey, in the film, *The Chapel of Sacred Mirrors* expressed that "A painting is a repository of consciousness."

Julia Cameron, author of *The Artist's Way,* stated "Art is a spiritual transaction." She mentions that artists are visionaries and art is an act of faith. Cameron says that the thought 'Creative dreams are egotistical' is something to clear from your mind. Piet Mondrian echoes Cameron's words in his statement "The position of the artist is humble. He is essentially a channel." Alex Grey adds "The artists take on the task of manifesting the unconscious world dream."

Invitation to expand:

How does a certain art form make you feel? What feelings does it evoke? What is its purpose for being on your wall, in your book, in your home? What art will you create today?

ASTROLOGY

"We are born at any given moment, in a given place and like vintage years of wine, we have the qualities of the year and of the season of which we are born. Astrology does not lay claim to anything more." Carl Jung

According to an article featured in the April 2009 issue of Natural Awakenings magazine, internationally renowned Astrologer, Shaman and author Michelle Karén, M.A., D.F. Astrol. S, shared that when Ancient Chaldean Priests studied the night, they noticed correlations between the planet positions and specific events and realized the same eclipses in the same sign created similar effects. From this, astrology, or the language of the stars was born (astro-logos: the language of the stars).

Karén stated that astrology's destiny was diverse and controversial. Many religions banned astrology fearing they would lose their power. It was also ridiculed because of misconceptions about free will. However, it survived and was studied by great minds including Galileo, Copernicus, Newton and Einstein.

She also stated that astrology is "A precious tool for personal empowerment. Based on the exact date, time and place of birth, it provides a precise map to every area of one's life and enables one to determine the successful date to launch any venture, whether buying a house, investing in or selling real estate or stocks, getting engaged or married."

Karén expressed that "The less we know about ourselves, the more enslavement we risk." With power and wisdom comes freedom. By understanding the strengths and weaknesses we entered this life with we are more capable of living our greatest potential. Karén mentioned that your life adventures are determined by your choices and how conscious you are of patterns revealed by your astrological chart.

Karén ends the article with these words: "If you re-discover the basic symbolism of the planets and signs by observing nature, you will realize there is a specific logic and wisdom to the "architecture of life." When you do not study your blue print given at birth, it is like driving around hoping to find the address you seek." Kindly visit Karén at www.michellekaren.com.

AYURVEDIC MEDICINE

According to the Merriam Webster medical dictionary, Ayurveda is "the traditional medicine of India, that preceded and evolved independently of Western medicine and integrates body, mind and spirit using a comprehensive holistic approach by emphasizing diet, herbal remedies, exercise, meditation, breathing and physical therapy." It is a 5,000 year old healing system and philosophy.

Dr. David Simon, best- selling author and co- founder of the Chopra Center once stated "The best use of a physician's knowledge is to teach patients how to heal themselves." He believed a true healer must be a diagnostician, medicine man, psychotherapist and an expert mind, physical body and spirit navigator.

According to Ayurvedic philosophy, 3 basic body/energy types or doshas (Kapha, Vata and Pitta) exist. Each type is to avoid certain foods. Kapha controls growth, supplies water to the body and maintains the immune system. In balance, kapha manifests as love and forgiveness while imbalance leads to insecurity and envy.

Vata controls bodily functions including blood circulation, breathing, blinking and heartbeat. With balanced vata, creativity and vitality is expressed. An imbalanced vata brings fear and anxiety.

Pitta controls metabolic systems, including digestion, absorption, nutrition and temperature. Balanced pitta leads to contentment and intelligence while imbalance leads to ulcers and anger.

You can be a mix of three doshas and dominance in one or two results in imbalance. The imbalance may be caused by stress, weather and diet. Ayurvedic philosophy embraces the five elements of space, air, earth, fire and water as comprising everything in the universe including the human body.

BEES

"Like the honeybee, the sage should gather wisdom from many scriptures."
Bhagavad Gita

In the documentary, *The Vanishing of the Bees,* the plight of the bees is examined. Since the days of Egypt, honeybees have been pollinating food. The honeybee has been the symbol of hard work, unity and cooperation. Scientist Dennis van Engelsdorp of Pen State University Dept. of Entomology, stated, "If we want a diet that is more than wheat, oats, corn and rice we need honeybees." Honeybees pollinate one in every three bites of our food.

In the U.S., bees pollinate 15 billion dollars' worth of food annually. According to U.S.D.A, in America, in 2011, commercial beekeepers lost an average of 36% of their hives to Colony Collapse Disorder (CCD). CCD killed thousands of bees throughout Australia, Italy, France, Germany, Spain and U.S. Henri Clement, UNAF President stated it well with the words: "The future of the bee, like water and energy will define the ability of man to live on the planet."

What can you do? Although bees vanishing may be dismal, in the U.S., New York, Seattle, San Francisco and Chicago legalized beekeeping. Daily, you vote at least three times with what you put into your mouth. Shopping at Farmers' Markets; purchasing local, organic food free of artificial colors, preservatives and additives; using natural, toxic free chemicals and planting gardens (even window gardens for city dwellers) are suggestions for living healthier and in tune with nature.

CHINESE MEDICINE/TRADITIONAL CHINESE MEDICINE (TCM)

As Ted Kaptchuk, O.M.D stated in *The Web That Has No Weaver,* "Chinese medicine is a coherent and independent system of thought that developed over two millennia. Based on ancient texts, it is the result of a continuous process of critical thinking, extensive clinical observation, testing as well as being rooted in philosophy, logic, sensibility and habits of a civilization foreign to our own."

Acupuncture is one modality of Traditional Chinese Medicine (TCM) that began thousands of years ago in China. The treatment is a holistic one, in other words, no one part is understood without its relation to the whole. It involves the insertion of fine needles into the skin, along 12 unseen energy meridians throughout the body. TCM treats physical and emotional, mental and psychological conditions that often result from blocks in the energy or 'chi' of the patient. Other TCM modalities include herbal medicine, moxabustion (burning the mugwort herb), tui na (massage); cupping, electro acupuncture, Qigong and gua sha ("scrape away fever" in Chinese).

Mike Lambert, acupuncturist and psychologist stated "The meridian energy lines in acupuncture are channels of photon energy, or chi and the acupuncture points along these lines are like 'junction boxes' where the flow can be affected and balanced." He saw energy build up at these junctions (as a ball of light).

In TCM, Qi and Yin/Yang theory are fundamental concepts (See chi/qi section above). According to Giovanni Maciocia in *The Foundations of Chinese Medicine,* "Yin and Yang are an alternation of two opposite stages in time; in its purest form, Yang is totally immaterial and corresponds to pure energy and Yin, in its densest form, is totally material and corresponds to matter." Yang becomes Yin and vice versa. Further examples are Yin is night, water and produces energy while yang is day, fire and produces form. Kaptchuk stated "For the Chinese, Qi is the pulsation of the cosmos itself, Qi is not so much a force added to lifeless matter but the state of being of any phenomenon."

A TCM practitioner studies everything about someone including their face, their walk, tone of voice, pulse and tongue. Two patients may present with the same complaint, i.e. back pain, yet will receive a different treatment as the diagnosis may have a different root cause. As in Ayurvedic medicine, the treatment is affected by many factors including the patient's constitution. Therefore, because many factors influence the energetic layers of a person, including hydration, nourishment (food, thoughts, etc.), it is important to abstain from drinking alcohol and eating greasy, fried heavy foods before and after treatment. Like everything in life, acupuncture is most effective when holding an open mind and a desire to improve one's health.

CHIROPRACTIC

According to www.chiropractic.org, the nervous system is the body's primary control mechanism. A chiropractor focuses on the nervous system's relationship with the spine. The spine allows for freedom of movement and houses and protects the spinal cord. When the spine's vertebrae are misaligned through trauma or repetitive injury, range of motion is limited and spinal nerves are compromised (subluxations). This may lead to pain, disability and a decrease in life quality. A chiropractor adjusts subluxations, allowing normal nerve expression. The body then restores itself to health.

According to sciencebase.com, spinal manipulation has been is use for thousands of years globally to fix health problems. Daniel D. Palmer developed the modern version in the nineteenth century.

Palmer's first patient was his deaf janitor who became deaf after a neck injury. Palmer claimed to 'click' a joint into place and the man's hearing returned. Palmer was jailed for practicing medicine without a license but his son took up chiropractic and it became popular.

Chiropractors "Consider the body to be like a living machine – if a joint is misaligned or damaged then the smooth running of the machine can be upset causing inflammation, pressure on nerves and subsequent medical problems." Chiropractors assess posture, joint mobility and lifestyle tracking restricted or excessive joint movement, especially in the spine.

THE TRUTH ABOUT CHOLESTEROL

According to Dr. Natasha Campbell-McBride, author of *Put Your Heart in Your Mouth*, cholesterol is not the evil thing we believe it to be. She stated "Our bodies are made out of billions of cells. Almost every cell produces cholesterol all the time during our lives. Every cell of every organ has cholesterol as part of its structure."

She stated that cholesterol and saturated fats make the cell walls firm (otherwise we would look like giant worms); cholesterol is needed for cell communication (proteins attach to cell walls with the help of cholesterol and saturated fats); about 25% of cholesterol is taken up by the brain and synapses (brain cells connecting) depend on cholesterol. Without cholesterol, the brain is unable to make "apolipoprotein E" needed for synapses. Also, endocrine glands (adrenals and sex glands) make steroid hormones. Steroid hormones like testosterone and progesterone are made from cholesterol. Therefore, Dr. Natasha concluded that without cholesterol, you would not be able to learn or remember anything or "have children because every sex hormone in our bodies is made from cholesterol."

Although the body produces cholesterol as needed, cholesterol rich foods help the body so it does not work as hard making its own. Dr. Natasha stated "When we eat more cholesterol, the body produces less; when we eat less cholesterol, the body produces more." Foods rich in cholesterol are (from highest to lowest) caviar, cod liver oil, fresh egg yolks, butter, cold water fish and shellfish like salmon, sardines, mackerel and lard.

YOUR GUT & YOUR HEALTH

What is Colon hydrotherapy?

According to Erin McGill, Certified Colon Therapist, "Colon hydrotherapy (or colonic) is the safe, gentle infusion of warm filtered water into the rectum without chemicals or drugs. The individual lies comfortably on a treatment table and the therapist gently inserts a small, sterilized speculum into the rectum. The therapist monitors the temperature and flow of water infused into and out of the colon (large intestine)."

SOUL INGREDIENTS

Why choose colon hydrotherapy?
Erin stated that "We experience better health and well- being when the colon is clean and functioning normally. When the colon is congested with waste, poisons back up into our system and pollute our inner environment. This is called autointoxication, or "self-poisoning." Autointoxication is considered the underlying cause of many degenerative diseases." Some of the symptoms of autointoxication include:

*Constipation or Diarrhea	*Food allergies
* Overweight/underweight	*Irritability
* Cellulite	*Low back pain
* Depression/Anxiety	*Skin problems
* Menstrual problems	*Candida/ Yeast problems
*Asthma/sinus problems	*Frequent headaches

Erin has been practicing colon therapy since 1996. She can be reached at (413) 586-6360; 68 Bradford St., Suite D in Northampton, MA 01060.

CRANIOSACRAL THERAPY

According to information from Upledger Institute International on www.upledger.com, Craniosacral therapy (CST) was developed by osteopathic physician John E. Upledger, following scientific studies from 1975 to 1983 at Michigan State University, where he was Professor of Biomechanics. CST is a gentle, hands-on way to evaluate and enhance the craniosacral system's functioning. The Craniosacral system is made up of membranes and cerebrospinal fluid surrounding and protecting the brain and spinal cord.

CYMATICS

"[Cymatics] is like a looking glass into a hidden world."
Evan Grant

In his TED 2009 talk in Oxford, Evan Grant stated that cymatics "Is the

182

PAGONA

process of visualizing sound by vibrating a medium such as sound or water."
Grant shared that everything gives out data whether it is a smell, a sound
or vibration. A CymaScope is used to scientifically observe cymatic patterns.
Cymatics can be used: as an art form, in healing and education, to study
dolphin language and recreate patterns of nature.

DEATH

"Wherever your path takes you, may all your deathbed wishes come
true and may you celebrate each and every one of them many long years
before your final breath." Gay Hendricks, Ph.D.

What is death? Many in the Western world fear death and do not
to think about it. Often, knowledge about death comes from parents or
loved ones who painted it as a mysterious enemy or ignored it. In *Emotional
Wellness,* Osho stated "Death is the disappearance of a false entity in you,
the ego. Death also happens in love on a smaller scale, in a partial way,
hence, the beauty of love. Sleep is a very tiny death. Death is a great sleep.
You fall back into the original unity of existence. Your body disappears into
the earth, your breath disappears into the air, your fire goes back to sun, and
your water to the oceans and your inner sky has a meeting with your outer
sky. How can one hate death?"

What happens after you die? Do you die? *In Conversations With God,
Book I,* Neale Donald Walsch shared "You never do die. Life is eternal. You
are immortal. You simply change form." If you are immortal and do not
die, only change form, what happens when your physical body is no longer
breathing or functioning? In *Conversations with God, Book III*, Neale Donald
Walsch stated "In the time after your "death" you may choose to have every
question you ever had answered and open yourself to new questions you
never dreamed existed. You may choose to experience Oneness with All That
Is and you will have a chance to decide what you wish to be, do and have
next."

*Meditations on Living, Dying and Loss: Ancient Knowledge for a
Modern World from the First Complete Translation of the Tibetan Book of
the Dead,* stated, "Death is the state when all the gross levels of energy and
consciousness have dissolved and only the subtle energies and consciousness

183

remain." According to Tibetan Buddhism, one's consciousness at death determines future existences. Hence, death holds a "mirror of past actions," or reflects negative and positive life actions to your eyes.

Invitation to expand:
When Steve Jobs was 17, he read a quote "If you live each day as if it was your last, someday you'll certainly be right." Daily, he looked in the mirror and asked himself: "If today were the last day of my life, would I want to do what I am about to do today?" Whenever he received a "No" for many days, Jobs knew he needed to change something. Remembering he'll be dead soon was, in his words "the most important tool I've ever encountered to help me make the big choices in life because almost everything – all external expectations, pride, fear of embarrassment or failure fall away in the face of death, leaving only what is important." What if you implemented his advice in your daily routine? How would it affect and change your life?

DIAMOND ALIGNMENT

Diamond Alignment is a high frequency energy transmission via one's personal computer. It was developed by Jacqueline Joy and her multidimensional friends over a 10 year period. It raises one's frequency in two 6 minute sessions daily. For more information, click on www.diamondalignment.com.

ESSENTIAL OILS

According to *The Reference Guide for Essential Oils*, by Connie and Alan Higley, "Essential oils were mankind's first medicine and are pure, therapeutic grade volatile liquids distilled from plants (including seeds, flowers, bark, etc.)." Essential oils are a form of aromatherapy. Examples include lavender oil, regarded as the "Swiss Army knife" of essential oils because of its usefulness in many conditions including burns and relaxation. Peppermint oil is often used for headaches while cinnamon oil helps relax tight muscles, ease painful joints and relieve menstrual cramps.

For thousands of years, Ancient Chinese and Egyptian civilizations used them. Essential oils can be taken orally, applied to the skin or mixed with carrier oil like olive or coconut oil and used for a range of symptoms including physical pain and anxiety. For more information, visit www.pagona.com and click Essential Oils.

FRACTAL/SACRED GEOMETRY

Gregg Braden, in his book, *Fractal Time: The Secret of 2012 and a New World Age,* mentioned a math professor at Yale University, Benoit Mandelbrot who developed a way to see the underlying structure of the world. Mandelbrot noticed that patterns within patterns makeup this world structure and coined it fractal geometry, also known as sacred geometry. Braden stated if you understand the pattern of an atom, you can understand the fractal pattern of the solar system and thus the galaxy.

According to Bruce Rawles, of www.geometrycode.com, sacred geometry is the belief that geometry, harmonics, math ratios are found everywhere in nature and reveals the nature of each form and its vibrational resonances. This principle of oneness underlying all geometry permeates the architecture of all form.

The 5 Platonic solids (Tetrahedron, Cube or (Hexahedron), Octahedron, Dodecahedron and Icosahedron) are ideal models of crystal patterns throughout the mineral world. To the Greeks, these solids symbolized fire, earth, air, spirit (or ether) and water.

The circle, the simplest form, expresses unity, completeness and integrity. Bruce stated that "Atoms, cells, seeds, planets, and globular star systems all echo the spherical paradigm of total inclusion, acceptance, simultaneous potential and fruition, the macrocosm and microcosm."

FRACTAL TIME

"Time cannot be absolutely defined and there is an inseparable relation between time and signal velocity (speed of a wave)."
Einstein

In Gregg Braden's book, *The Secret of 2012 and a New World Age*, he mentioned the concept of fractal time. He stated "A growing body of evidence suggests that time's waves and the history within them, repeat as cycles within cycles. As each new cycle begins, it carries the same conditions as the past but with greater intensity. It's this fractal time that becomes the events of the universe and life."

Gregg Braden shared that the Mayans charted this fractal time on series of calendars. They understood the cycles and that we approached the end of the world age or cycle of 5,125 years. Ancient civilizations divide 25,625 year orbit (often rounded to 26,000) through the zodiac's 12 constellations into 5 world ages, each 5,125 years long. This 5,125 year cycle we are in ended on the winter solstice- 21 December 2012. The last humans to experience the shift from one world age to another lived in 3114 B.C., about 1,800 years before Moses.

What does this mean? Gregg Braden stated that 21 December 2012 was "A rare and powerful window of opportunity for our collective emergence into our greatest potential." On 21 December 2012, the solar system aligned with Milky Way's core and reset the calendar and a new world age began. In another 26,000 years, this will occur again.

The Hopi see this period as a time of "purification" occurring before the Earth's cleansing. As humanity moves from the end of a 26,000 year cycle into a new world age, humanity has the potential to move beyond limited thinking into greater expansion of all mental faculties. Every step you take has profound implications, especially for the old souls on the planet. You light the way to greater consciousness, worldwide peace and healing, shifting Gaia's vibration and everything contained within and outside it.

GEMSTONE/CRYSTAL THERAPY

According to Allison Hayes, "The Rock Girl", stones/crystals are living things that carry energy and that energy can be harnessed. They can be used to manifest abundance of love, money, health or whatever you desire. Allison suggested choosing stones specific to the desire. For example, you would choose rose quartz with citrine (makes things happen quickly) to manifest love quickly.

GUT AND PSYCHOLOGY SYNDROME (GAPS)

"The primary seat of insanity generally is in the region of the stomach and intestines."
Phillipe Pinel (1745-1828), French psychiatrist

Dr. Natasha Campbell-McBride developed the *Gut and Psychology Syndrome* (GAPS) protocol after successfully treating her autistic son with this. She largely based her work on the Specific Carbohydrate Diet (SCD) making necessary alterations. For more information, see Elaine Gottschall's book, *Breaking The Vicious Cycle, Intestinal Health Through Diet*.

In her book, *Gut and Psychology Syndrome*, Dr. Natasha Campbell-McBride stated that your body is inhabited by large numbers of micro-creatures. She explained that "The largest colonies of microbes live in our digestive system. A healthy adult, on average, carries 1.5-2 kg of bacteria in the gut."

The GAPS lifestyle is an anti-inflammatory diet built around healthy fat sources, vegetables and fruits and raw nuts and seeds. The protocol focuses on 3 principles. The first principle is to heal the gut by avoiding sugar and processed foods. Secondly, the gut is inoculated with beneficial microorganisms of high quality probiotics and fermented foods (amasi, kimchee, yogurt, coconut kefir and homemade sauerkraut). Amasi is native to Africa and considered one of the best probiotics. The third principle focuses on waste detoxification by toxin avoidance and detox strategies. One strategy includes drinking fresh vegetable juices to help purify blood and remove toxins. The foods in the GAPS diet may be modified according to the severity and condition treated.

What are the symptoms of a GAPS patient? In a GAPS patient, low numbers of beneficial bacteria, opportunistic and pathogenic microbes take over the digestive system, resulting in a constant production of toxicity from the gut to the brain. Dr. Natasha stated, "This is the toxicity which is probably making these adults and children autistic, schizophrenic, hyperactive, dyspraxic, dyslexic, psychotic, depressed, obsessed, etc."

She found that conditions including: A.D.D., A.D.H.D., autism, depression, dyslexia, dyspraxia and schizophrenia resolved or symptoms decreased once

187

a patient followed the set diet and protocol (GAPS). Although it may not be easy, if the family is involved and committed, wonderful results are seen in those dedicated to improving their health.

HADO MEDICINE

In his book, *The Secret Life of Water*, Masaru Emoto described Hado medicine. This modality focuses on the root cause of the illness, specifically the vibration of the illness. Once the frequency of the illness is known, the exact opposite wavelength can overlap the illness's wavelength and the illness vanishes. A form of Hado medicine is flower essences, developed by Dr. Edward Bach. The energy of the vibration of the flowers is transferred to water. When you drink this water, you receive physical and mental benefits.

HEB (HIGHLY EVOLVED BEINGS)

In *Conversations with God, Book III,* Neal Donald Walsch stated that highly evolved beings (HEB) live in nature, communicating telepathically while living in unity understanding all are interrelated. They do not kill and divide their natural resources equally. In their societies, they live by two principles "We Are All One" and "There's enough." What is valued is "that which produces benefit to all." The elders are responsible for organizing and supervising caring, education, housing and feeding. "Their whole beingness comes from "what is so" and "what works."

Neale Donald Walsch tells you that in HEB societies "There are no governments as you would understand them and no laws. There are councils usually of elders. There are what could be best translated into your language as "mutual agreements." These have been reduced to a Triangular Code: Awareness, Honesty, and Responsibility." They know they live forever; it's a matter of what form they will take. They choose what they would like to learn and acknowledge all they see.

Invitation to expand:
Whether you embrace the concept of HEBs or not, much can be learned

by embracing their code of Awareness, Honesty and Responsibility. Imagine what the world would look like, the depth of your relationships and everything in your life if you followed this code.

HERBAL MEDICINE

According to the National Herbalist Association of Australia, "Herbal medicine is the oldest and most widely used system of medicine in the world today. It is medicine made exclusively from plants and is used in all societies and is common to all cultures."

In TCM, herbal medicine is an important tool that treats many conditions. Herbs are classified according to certain properties such as: bitter, sweet, warming, cooling, neutral, salty, aromatic as well as what conditions they treat. Herbs may be prescribed in their raw state to be made into a tea or taken in capsules or mixed with other herbs in a formula.

HOMEOPATHY

German Physician Dr. Samuel Hahnemann developed homeopathy when he noticed that the essence of the bark of the cinchona salisaya used to treat malaria, caused malaria symptoms when taken orally. According to the Society of Homeopaths, homeopathy treats the person with highly diluted non-toxic substances, mainly in pill form to trigger the body's natural system of healing. It is based on treating 'like with like', thus, a substance that causes symptoms in large doses, can be used in small amounts to treat those same symptoms. For example, drinking too much coffee can cause sleeplessness and agitation, thus, according to this principle, when made into a homeopathic medicine, it may treat people with these symptoms.

HYDROTHERAPY

One form of hydrotherapy- colon hydrotherapy was discussed. Below I mention one technique of exposure to steam baths to help detox and increase skin's perspiration.

In *Energy Secrets*, Alla Svirinskaya mentioned the healing power of a traditional Russian banya, an ancient steam bath using wet heat involving exposure to heat, cold and rest. This was believed to flush away sins and researchers found it helps normalize blood pressure and helps with diabetes, kidney and metabolic conditions.

As banyas are difficult to find in the West, you may replicate the technique by following these steps: Enter a sauna/steam room between 9 am- 11 am with dry skin having eaten a small breakfast. Cover head with a towel and ensure your feet are warm. Next, while breathing through your nose, sit and relax for 5 minutes. (Leave when you begin to sweat). Dry your body and lie down and rest 5 minutes before returning to sauna for 10 minutes. Repeat these steps and drink tiny sips of water, mint tea or combination of carrot, black radish and beetroot juice with honey (juice is full of vitamins and minerals). To make beetroot juice, Alla suggested peeling, cutting it in half and soaking ingredients (carrot and black radish) 3-4 hours before juicing. Now return to the sauna for the last time, remaining longer and then following it with a cold shower or cold pool. Rest for 30 minutes before enjoying a massage.

Two more warm hydrotherapy options include Epsom salt and aromatherapy baths. The Epsom salt bath encourages toxin elimination. Soak in hot bath of 225-440 g Epsom salt. When you exit the bath, dry your skin and go to bed, ensuring that you rinse and moisturize your skin the next morning.

For the aromatherapy bath, add desired essential oils, using 5-10 drops into the bath, relaxing 20 minutes. You may wish to use frankincense, cedarwood or lavender essential oils. Frankincense purifies and relaxes, cedarwood eliminates toxins and lavender is good for anxiety, worry and wounds.

In the article entitled *Researching the Experiential Effects of Applied Cymatics in Water for Healing Purposes Using Crystal Bowls Tuned to the Harmonic Solfeggio Scale,* Aliza Hava stated that hydrotherapy and new water healing techniques treat many medical conditions. Techniques such as Watsu, Jahara, Water Dance and Hydrotherapy for the disabled are gaining momentum worldwide, especially in Israel. Amita Media and Shai Danon, founders of www.Ahava528.com, combined "Three aspects of science into one technique: Directing accurate sound waves to energy centers of the body, utilizing water as the best known conductor and Quartz Crystal as the best naturally transmitting amplifier." They worked with over 30 hydrotherapists and acknowledge the impact these sounds have on patient's recovery.

HYPNOTHERAPY

According to The National Board for Certified Clinical Hypnotherapists, (NBCCH, Inc.) hypnosis is a state of inward attention and focused concentration, often called a trance or altered state of consciousness. With a concentrated and focused mind, you are better able to use your inner power, make changes and live a better life. Hypnosis and self-hypnosis allow you to use more of your potential and gain more self-control.

NBCCH stated that hypnotherapy is useful for conditions including: addictions, allergies, anxiety, concentration, skin problems, weight management, depression, gastrointestinal issues, phobias, stress management, pain, nausea relief and childbirth.

IRIDOLOGY

According to the International Iridology Practitioners Association, iridology is "The study of the iris, (colored part), of the eye. This structure identifies how our body reacts to our environment and what symptoms to expect and where we may have problems with age. It helps identify inherited emotional patterns, which can create or maintain physical symptoms, as well as our lessons, challenges and gifts or talents."

LIGHT THERAPY (PHOTOTHERAPY)

According to the www.mayoclinic.com, light therapy treats seasonal affective disorder (SAD) or depression that occurs at certain times each year, by exposure to artificial light. During light therapy, you sit or work near a light therapy box that mimics natural outdoor light. Light therapy is thought to affect brain chemicals linked to mood, easing SAD symptoms.

Conditions that light therapy treats include: seasonal affective disorder (SAD), non seasonal depression or insomnia and skin conditions including psoriasis (using UV light). It is also being studied as a treatment for conditions, including: obsessive-compulsive disorders, jet lag, sleep disorders, Parkinson's disease, dementia and Attention-deficit hyperactivity disorder (ADHD).

LOGOTHERAPY

Dr. Viktor Frankl, a psychiatrist and prisoner number 119,104, founded logotherapy, or existential analysis. Logotherapy's foundation of existential analysis or finding meaning in one's life is the motivating factor that drives one's life. Logotherapy transformed Dr. Frankl while he was in the Nazi concentration camp. In *Man's Search for Meaning,* Frankl described a life transforming day:

"I became disgusted with the state of affairs which compelled me, daily and hourly, to think of only trivial things. I forced my thoughts to turn to another subject. Suddenly I saw myself standing on the platform of a well-lit, warm and pleasant lecture room. In front of me sat an attentive audience on comfortable upholstered seats. I was giving a lecture on the psychology of the concentration camp! All that oppressed me at that moment became objective, seen and described from the remote viewpoint of science. By this method I succeeded somehow in rising above the situation, above the sufferings of the moment and I observed them as if they were already of the past. Both I and my troubles became the object of an interesting psycho-scientific study undertaken by myself. What does Spinoza say in his Ethics? Emotion, which is suffering, ceases to be suffering as soon as we form a clear picture of it."

Dr. Frankl's search for meaning helped him rise above the horrific conditions in the concentration camp. He learned that true salvation comes from creating meaning in life. Dr. Frankl realized he is the author of his emotions and his thoughts. What meaning do you give your life? How do you create meaning in your world?

MAGNETIC HEALING

This Japanese healing system is based on the fact that all matter is made up of energy. Therefore, the electromagnetic fields created by strong magnets can be used to balance the energy of the diseased body.

"A negative magnetic field can function like an antibiotic to help destroy bacterial, fungal and viral infections by promoting oxygenation and lowering the body's acidity." William H. Philpott, M.D.

MASSAGE THERAPY

"For rubbing can bind a joint that is too loose, and loosen a joint that is too rigid."
Hippocrates, "Father of Modern Medicine"

Massage has been used around the world for thousands of years to release pain and blocks (physical, emotional) from the body. Examples of massage include: The Arvigo Techniques of Maya Abdominal Therapy™; tui na (China), kunye (Tibet and Himalayas) which regards illness and treatment as comprised of 5 elements (earth, water, fire, metal and air); lomi-lomi (Hawaii) and Shiatsu (finger and palm pressure, stretches and other techniques).

The Arvigo Techniques of Maya Abdominal Therapy™ are based on uterine massage developed by Dr. Rosita Arvigo while she studied with Mayan healer and Belize's renowned Shaman, Don Elijio Panti. It repositions displaced uterine organs that restrict chi, blood and lymph flow. This massage can be performed on males and includes herbology, nutrition, massage, anatomy, physiology and emotional spiritual healing. For more information, visit www. arvigotherapy.com.

MATRIX ENERGETICS

Matrix Energetics was developed by Dr. Richard Bartlett, DC, ND and described as "The science and art of transformation." It is a consciousness technology incorporating intention, letting go, quantum physics, string theory and Sheldrake's concept of morphic field. According to Sheldrake, a morphic field includes morphogenetic, behavioral, social, cultural and mental fields. It is a "Universal database for organic (living) and abstract (mental) forms that organizes the field's structure and activity patterns at all levels of complexity."

Dr. Bartlett describes Matrix Energetics in many ways, one of which is "Universal transcendent awareness that is spreading." You let go of your left brain, allow yourself to play and drop into your heart center, allowing for possibilities previously unknown, to occur. While participating in the seminar, my consciousness shifted to an increased and heightened sense of possibilities and an increase in clairvoyance. It is an experience that stays with you and one I highly recommend to all.

In his book, *The Physics of Miracles: tapping into the field of consciousness potential,* Dr. Bartlett stated that the secret to manifestation is stepping into a unified field of consciousness. When you tap into the morphic field of Matrix Energetics, you tap into a huge unified field of consciousness and amplify your power. It is in this space that your reality changes.

MULTIVARIATE RESONANCE TECHNOLOGY/ OmHARMONICS

"Multivariate Resonance Technology is a proprietary sequencing of sound frequencies carefully sculpted to stimulate, balance and activate the four holistic intelligences."

This audio meditation technology or OmHarmonics, uses binaural beat patterns to allow you to meditate instantly and can be listened to for 15-30 minutes daily. You listen to it before an exam, while traveling on a plane, at bedtime to help you sleep or anytime you would like to relax.

According to information obtained from www.omharmonics.com, OmHarmonics stimulates the following four holistic intelligences: physical, emotional, mental and spiritual. Physical Intelligence is connected to heart beat regulation and breathing frequencies and facilitates mind clearing. Emotional Intelligence is connected to heart beat and heart coherence frequencies and stimulates the emotions of gratitude, love and forgiveness. The binaural frequencies of alpha and theta brainwave ranges are connected to mental intelligence and allow for expansion of an open mind. Spiritual Intelligence comes from specific light spectra frequencies that translate sound vibration.

NATUROPATHIC MEDICINE

According to the American Association of Naturopathic Physicians, naturopathic medicine is "Steeped in traditional healing methods, principles and practices. Naturopathic medicine focuses on holistic, proactive prevention and comprehensive diagnosis and treatment." Naturopaths use protocols that minimize harm, therefore facilitating the body's innate ability to restore and maintain health.

Naturopathic students, in their four year training, complete science courses including human anatomy and physiology, biochemistry, embryology, histology, pathology and neuroscience. They study concepts such as naturopathic clinical theory and counseling, food and dietary systems, botanical medicine, hydrotherapy and homeopathy; case analysis and management and medical specialties such as pediatrics, neurology, public health, dermatology and gastroenterology.

Many people confuse naturopathic and osteopathic medicine. Naturopathic Doctors (ND) emphasize preventive medicine and supportive care for patients with AIDS, cancer and other illnesses. They complete 1,000+ hours of clinical training in naturopathic clinics and offices.

In contrast, Doctors of Osteopathic (D.O.) "Have nearly 14,000 hours of supervised clinical training behind them," noted David Walls, executive director of Osteopathic Physicians and Surgeons of Oregon (OPSO). Naturopathic students encounter less variety of diseases and disorders than osteopathic students trained in hospitals.

NUMEROLOGY

"To study the vibratory value of numbers and letters is to study the divine creative energies in various degrees of manifestation."
Faith Javane and Dusty Bunker

According to Faith Javane and Dusty Bunker, authors of *Numerology and the Divine Triangle*, numbers "represent universal principles through which all things evolve and continue to grow in cyclic fashion." Numbers 1- 9 symbolize the stages an idea undergoes before it becomes reality. According to the authors, these stages result in all manifestation.

Javane and Bunker state that you have four personal numbers at birth which indicate life lessons to learn and show spiritual growth you may experience. The numbers in your birthdate and the letters in your name determine these four personal numbers. These numbers are: Life Lesson Number, Soul Number, Outer Personality Number and Path of Destiny Number. The Outer Personality Number indicates how you appear to others; The Life Lesson Number speaks about life lessons to learn while the Soul Number asks what does your inner desire yearn to be. Lastly, the Path of Destiny Number represents what you came to accomplish in this lifetime.

OSTEOPATHIC MEDICINE

According to the American Association of Colleges of Osteopathic Medicine, "osteopathic medicine is a distinct form of medical practice in the United States. It provides modern medicine including prescription drugs, surgery, and technology to diagnose disease and evaluate injury by emphasizing health promotion and disease prevention."

Osteopathic doctors (DO), view the patient holistically, integrating physical, psychological and social needs. DOs learn that structure influences function. Therefore, if there is a problem in one area of the body's structure, function in that and other areas may be affected.

PAST LIFE REGRESSION

According to Monica Hoffman, past life regressionist, www. pastLIFEregression.NYC.com, many people have misconceptions about this healing modality. She mentions these below.

"Many benefits exist and of course, Past Life Regression may stir a fear of information revealed. It may demonstrate a responsibility to take ownership of undesirable patterns and circumstances. Even when one is not at fault, he/she knows deeper psyche changes can be made. When these changes occur, our circumstances and world around us also change."

Many do not choose Past Life Regression because of 4 misconceptions:

1. "I don't want to be in a trance where I may not have control." Past Life Regression is not done in a trance-state with no control over self. It is similar to guided meditation. You are aware, yet, extremely relaxed in a clear, focused state of mind.

2. "You cannot hypnotize me." This is somewhat true. If you do not trust the healing process and professional, it will not work. If a professional does not feel right, trust your feelings, remembering other qualified professionals exist.

3. "What if I am imagining this past life?" Your memory can recall many details. Whether they occurred or did not occur, according to your recollection, is not important. You have your perceptions and experiences. What is important is retrieving patterns to explain and resolve the present time.

4. "I do not want to re-experience anything bad." A trauma does not need to be relived. A Past Life Regressionist reminds you to 'float above the scene' to not re-experience unpleasantness. Once your left, logical brain understands what occurred in the past and how it affects the present and future, the negative experiences dissolve.

For you to heal, you must be willing to heal. When you are receptive to knowing missing components of your life's mystery, you gain awareness. With awareness, you navigate through life more successfully. Profound invincibility is realized when you understand how you survived the unthinkable in history. Also, upon realizing your spirit, through time and space, is physical, then non-physical and physical again, your consciousness expands and you are ready for greatness!"

PARALLEL UNIVERSE

"We all exist in multiple universes and create our own bubble of reality."
Gerald O'Donnell, leading expert in military science of Remote Viewing

According to Burt Goldman of www.quantumjumping.com, physicist Alan Guth came up with a parallel universes theory or inflationary theory of cosmology based on many observations. Professor Guth is a Professor of Physics at Massachusetts Institute of Technology (M.I.T). Many of his peers believe his theory that when the universe began, instead of gravity keeping things together, a reverse gravitation repelled everything from it. He called this reverse gravitation a "false vacuum."

Another part to Professor Guth's theory states that at the big bang, this "false vacuum" decayed and created vast numbers of particles. These particles are the same as those that began our universe. According to this theory, the universe is larger than predicted and these particles originated as the decay became bubbles. If true, this theory proves many universes exist with the same properties and laws of physics.

What do these different universes contain? Two ideas help explain this. The first is that the universes are the same in matter and physical laws as our universe (belief in parallel universes). One exception is a different element in their creation, allowing these other worlds the potential to have every possible and available particle combination. In other words, they would operate by the same principles but with every possible combination. For example, the oceans would exist where our continents are and vice versa. The second idea is that other worlds are different because they do not operate in 3 D as our universe does.

The first concept- parallel universes, allows for the idea that you exist at the same time in more than one place. Traveling to these universes, you could 'meet' your other selves. Imagine the unlimited possibilities if your individual beings could meet and transfer knowledge and intelligence. In one world you could be a farmer and in another world a healer. With quantum jumping, Burt Goldman, shows you how to do that. According to Goldman, quantum jumping allows you to visualize and communicate with yourself in parallel universes. He states it is the result of 31 years of study in areas including yoga, meditation and remote viewing.

PSYCHO-CYBERNETICS

According to Dr. Maxwell Maltz, author of *The New Psycho-Cybernetics*, Psycho-Cybernetics is a collection of principles, insights and methods that allow you to analyze the contents of your self-image; identify incorrect self-image programming and change it as well as use your imagination to reprogram your self-image and move you toward your goals. Albert Einstein practiced Psycho-Cybernetics as well as many successful leaders.

"Human beings always act and feel and perform in accordance with what they imagine to be true about themselves and their environment."

This, according to Psycho-Cybernetics, is the book's most important information. As mentioned earlier, what you do not know, you are unable to change. When you analyze something, uncover the truth about yourself, you can alter it. Otherwise, you remain not in a state of awareness but in ignorance.

PSYCHOMETRY

"In psychometry, a person holds an object and is impressed with feelings or visions about the person to whom the object belongs. Everyone and every object have energy and the vibrations of an object often reveal the history of its owner. Psychometry is used a lot in criminal investigations."
James Van Praagh, spiritual medium

QUANTUM ACTIVATORS

"Quantum Activators are artworks created by Andre Ferrella that manipulate light, esoteric shapes and ethereal colors to stimulate the visual cortex, activating the pineal gland to calibrate our DNA and raise our multidimensional frequencies."
Andre Ferrella, Artist of the Spirit, www.livingmuseum.com.

Artist of the Spirit, Andre Ferrella shares that quantum activators increase your connection to Oneness allowing you to remember on a quantum, multidimensional level. Simply standing in front of a quantum activator for 5 minutes allows you to experience many enlightening things. My profoundly enriching and ethereal experience with one of his quantum activators often brings a smile to my soul.

QUANTUM PHYSICS/QUANTUM THEORY

"Quantum physics has found that there is no empty space in the human cell, but it is a teeming, electric-magnetic field of possibility or potential." Dr. Deepak Chopra

What is quantum physics? According to www.thefreedictionary.com, quantum means:

"1. A quantity or amount.
2. Something that can be counted or measured.
3. Physics
    a. The smallest amount of a physical quantity that can exist independently, especially a discrete quantity of electromagnetic radiation."

When applied to physics, quantum means: 1. (Physics / Atomic Physics)
    a. the smallest quantity of some physical property, such as energy, a system can possess according to the quantum theory
    b. a particle with such a unit of energy"

Hence, quantum physics is the study of energy units that cannot be divided, as described in quantum theory. According to John Gribbin's book *In Search of Schrodinger's Cat*, quantum theory incorporates the following 5 ideas: 1) Energy is not continuous, but comes in small but discrete units. 2) These particles behave like particles and waves. 3) The movement of these particles is random. 4) It is impossible to know the position and momentum of a particle at the same time. The more precisely one is known, the less precise the measurement of the other is. 5) The atomic world is unlike the world we live in.

Dr. John F. Demartini shared that "Quantum physicists now know that all subatomic particles such as protons, electrons, neutrons, quarks and mesons are all actually waves."

Author and physicist Dr. Fred Alan Wolf expressed, "Today, probably more than in any other day, we're facing a revolution in our thinking about the physical universe-the stuff that you and I are made of. This revolution, brought to a head by the discoveries of new physics, including relativity and quantum mechanics, appears to reach well beyond our preconceived vision that is based on the concept of concrete solid reality."

[I can't accept quantum mechanics because] "I like to think the moon is there even if I am not looking at it."
Albert Einstein

Invitation to expand:
Think about what you were taught about the Universe, protons, electrons, etc. Have your views changed? Why or why not?

REFLEXOLOGY

The Reflexology Association of Canada defines reflexology as: "A natural healing art based on the principle that there are reflexes in the feet, hands and ears and their referral areas which correspond to every part, gland and organ of the body. Through application of pressure on these reflexes without tools or lotions, the feet being the primary area of application, reflexology relieves tension, improves circulation and helps promote the natural function of the related areas of the body."

REIKI

According to *The Power to Heal*, Robert Pellegrino-Estrich stated that reiki is: "manually applied energy directly to the body. It is a direct transfer of universal energy from and through the therapist to the client." Many variations of Reiki exist and can be learned from a Reiki Master.

TAOIST PHILOSOPHY

"Taoists regard the soles of the feet as the roots of the body and the root is important as the foundation for the work of the spirit body."
Mantak Chia

According to Mantak Chia, founder of the Universal Healing Tao System and author of 25 books, traditional Taoist meditation enables men and women to reach a state of healing love. For women, this is obtained through cultivation, transformation and circulation of sexual energy, or jing. Jing is a generative, creative energy needed for chi (vital life force) and shen (spiritual energy) development.

In his book, *Healing Love through the Tao,* Mantak mentioned that Taoist meditation views the body as comprised of 3 parts: physical body, soul body and spirit body. Each of these is equally important and the goal of Taoist meditation is to give birth to the self. Giving birth to self is "Awakening the part of oneself that perceives and acts free of the boundaries of environmental education and karmic conditioning."

THOUGHT FIELD THERAPY (TFT)

"When I observe a number of suffering patients who did not respond to our usual treatment modalities, suddenly get better after TFT algorithms are given, I don't need a double-blind controlled study to tell me the value of TFT."
James McCoy, MD Chief, Pain Clinic, Hematology Service,
Assistant Chief, Neuroscience Department

Callahan Techniques® Thought Field Therapy (TFT) was founded and co- developed by Roger J. Callahan, Ph.D., clinical psychologist and his wife Joanne M. Callahan. According to www.rogercallahan.com, "TFT is the origin of meridian tapping therapy that uses nature's healing system to balance the body's energy system and an alternative to long term or drug related psychotherapy." It is a quick and painless self- help tool using a tapping sequence (a healing code) to balance the body's energy.

Cary Graig, a Stanford engineering graduate and ordained minister, took the knowledge of Dr. Roger Callahan's TFT and developed Emotional Freedom Technique (EFT). EFT is similar to TFT and also involves tapping various acupuncture meridian points while repeating certain statements.

According to www.tapping.com, "Tapping is a simple but effective technique somewhere in between hypnosis, meditation and acupressure." You can learn it in minutes and apply instant relief to stressful situations. Meridian tapping may help with: anger management, insomnia, physical and emotional pain, procrastination and stress relief. It is something I often teach my clients.

TIBETAN MEDICINE

According to Eliot Tokar, Tibetan medical practitioner since 1983 (www. tibetanmedicine.com), Tibetan medicine defines three main systems that control the body's processes, called humors. These humors are created at different developmental stages in the womb by 5 elements (Earth, Water, Fire, Wind and Space) interacting with your mind's developmental process.

"Embryologically, the mind acts as the basis for the creation of each individual's 3 principle physical systems of Wind, Bile and Phlegm. These three systems create and sustain the body's functions."

Wind creates many functions including circulation of blood, thoughts and food. Wind may manifest as the mind expressed as attachment or desire and a materialist world view.

Bile controls functions such as metabolism, liver function, vision and allows your mind to function discriminately. Bile may manifest as aggression, hatred and anger.

Phlegm creates the physical principle of energy creating will and function and provides the body's lubrication. Phlegm manifests as ignorance or incomprehension.

A disturbance (from diet, behavior or environment) in one or a combination of these principle systems results in illness. How the above factors result in illness depends on whether the problem is acute or chronic. Tibetan medicine, like Chinese medicine, views illness as individual and bases it on each patient's situation and background.

TONING

"Nature and Grace - the physical and the spiritual - reflect each other and reveal "the great fact" that there is a secret tone scale - or set of sounds - that vibrates at the exact

frequencies required to transform spirit to matter or matter to spirit."
Leonard G. Horowitz, M.D,
author of *Healing Codes for the Biological Apocalypse*

"When we do toning, drumming, chanting, or tuning forks – it can be a way to direct energy for transformational purposes." David Hulse, D.D.

According to information on www.kryon.com, Dr. Todd Ovokaitys stated that The Pineal Toning Technique™ uses sound (tones) and specific sequenced syllables and includes 24 levels. Dr. Todd experienced specific tones that were shown to him.

According to Kryon "Humans typically operate on 4 of 12 strands of DNA, leaving 8 strands (higher dimensions) non-operational or blocked. The tones seem to be a catalyst for unblocking the filter/s extending into the other 8 DNA strands." These tones can activate the dormant DNA strands/layers causing relaxation and many mind expansive experiences.

Dr. Todd stated that it is now known that the pineal gland secretes melatonin and maintains serotonin levels. It is located in the center of the brain between the left and right hemispheres. Light also influences this gland, which is also referred to as the center of the soul or a spiritual gateway.

Pineal toning is a powerful and easy to learn self- healing tool. These tones had a profound effect on my ability to see beyond 3D. Many sensations and colors were noted and I revel in this whenever I sing them. Every experience is different and unique to the individual.

VIBRATIONAL MEDICINE

"Everything in the body is reflected in the energy field. There is a group of cells in the body, which came out of phase with the others, then the negative energy in that portion of the field creates a resistance to the hand's movement above the body and the healer knows he reached the source of the problem in the body."
Colin Lambert, New Zealand healer for 30+ years

According to Kryon, 11 aspects of vibrational medicine exist. These concepts are: Phototherapy, *color therapy, *homeopathy, sound therapy, spiritual healing, *mind/body medicine, *acupuncture, magnetic therapy, *crystals, gems and rocks and electromedicine. (*Please reference individual sections).

Richard Gerber, MD, author of *Vibrational Medicine,* shared his definition of vibrational medicine in an interview with Edward Brown. "Vibrational medicine is a diagnostic and healing approach to illness using energy in various forms and frequencies. As a therapy, vibrational medicine is the application of different types of energy for healing, including approaches as traditional as X-ray and radiation therapy for cancer, the use of electrical nerve stimulation for treating pain and electromagnetic field stimulators for accelerating the healing of fractured bones. Full spectrum light is used for treating seasonal affective disorders or the 'winter blues'. However, vibrational medicine also covers the more subtle forms of treatment such as acupuncture, homeopathy, flower essences, therapeutic touch. The latter involve using subtle life-force medicine but they are energetic therapies nonetheless. This is the spectrum from the more traditional to a range of therapies that stress treatment of the whole person, sometimes referred to as 'complementary' medicine."

Dr. Gerber explained that vibrational practitioners influence the individual's consciousness, helping gain insight into predisposing factors creating their illness, or why the illness crystallized at this time.

The vibrational approach, especially the subtle energy medicine approach, injects selective energy frequencies in the body that encourage the body's self-healing systems to do the work. Some of the most elegant approaches for healing cancer and AIDS may involve using selective energy frequencies or electromagnetic fields. There are indications this technology has been around but was suppressed.

Dr. Gerber stated that assessing the acupuncture meridian system can help detect disturbances in the etheric body before they manifest in physical form. If this becomes reality, a new level of preventive medicine will be birthed. He stated, "The acupuncture meridian system appears to be the interface between the physical body and the higher energy control systems."

Vibrational medicine is the first scientific approach that integrates science and spirituality. By viewing the body as a multi-dimensional energy system we approach how the soul manifests through molecular biology. Various people doing past life regression are envisioning the soul's progress through life and illness as an expression of obstacles the soul is trying to overcome while learning. How karma fits into this is an individualized thing.

YOGA

"All types of energy have one common factor: they vibrate. This vibration is called nada or nadam, cosmic music. Plato called it the "music of the spheres", the music of Nature, known as OM. It is the voice of silence. OM is the eternal name of Absolute consciousness, I-AM. OM is the home of the entire existence. OM is the seed and essence of all existence. OM (A-U-M) is a mixture of: "A" manifestation, "U" growth, "M" perfection, completion."
Shri Brahmananda Sarasvati

Yoga is a mental, physical and spiritual discipline that originated in India. Yoga is a Sanskrit word meaning "union"- "uniting self with the universe." When you practice yoga, your focus is higher consciousness. According to Alex Grey, "The goal of yoga is to unite you with God."

Forms of yoga include: Bhakti, Bikram, Kriya, Laughter yoga and Jivamukti yoga. Each emphasizes different techniques.

Bikram Yoga is a series of 26 Hatha Yoga postures and two Pranayama breathing exercises that are done in a hot room for 90 minutes. Bikram yoga works every muscle, tendon, ligament, joint and internal organ in the body.

Jivamukti Yoga "Samadhi is a trance state in which the separation between the yogini, the practice of Yoga and concentration merge into one, a state of bliss." Each class has a theme, incorporating yoga scripture, chanting, meditation, asana (postures), pranayama and music.

Kriya Yoga is a scientific technique of meditation for attaining direct personal experience of God. This was taught to Mahatma Gandhi, Elijah and Jesus.

Laughter Yoga (according to www.laughteryoga.org) "combines unconditional laughter with yogic breathing (pranayama)." Its founder, Dr. Madan Kataria, launched it in 1995 and today, it is global with 6000+ Laughter Clubs in 60 countries. Laughter yoga is based on science stating the body cannot differentiate between fake and real laughter. Therefore, the same physiological and psychological benefits are obtained.

ZAGOVOR
(Russian Chanting Technique)

International renowned healer, Alla Svirinskaya, in her book *Energy Secrets: The Ultimate Well-Being Plan,* discusses zagovor or Russian Chanting Technique. She shared that healing techniques evolved around words, whispering spells and chants with herbs or other healing modalities. In Russia, a spell, "a form of psychotherapeutic suggestion or powerful affirmation of intent put into words" is called zagovor.

Alla stated that zagovor is done one to one, away from others, using a low, rhythmical, monotonous voice. It works because it appeals to the right and left sides of the brain, activating the right hemisphere by building images and using affirmations to activate the left side of the brain. As an example, Alla mentioned a technique she uses with patients. They imagine their hands are very cold while imagining their feet are very hot. This, she says, engages the brain in two different tasks simultaneously.

ZUMBA

According to www.zumba.com, zumba is a Latin-inspired dance-fitness program blending international music and contagious steps to form an addictive "fitness-party." It began in 2001 and is the world's largest dance-fitness program in more than 125 countries.

Alberto "Beto" Perez, from Colombia, created the Zumba experience after he forgot his music while teaching aerobics. He used his mix of salsa and merengue and his class loved it and zumba was born.

SOUL INGREDIENTS

My wish for you:

I leave you with a message I emailed my three sisters after my last grandparent died in 2011. "May your 86,400 daily seconds be filled with love, absolute presence and greatness. May every thought bring clarity; your arms embrace hundreds and your minds understand yourselves and a million others. May each seed you plant fall on open ears; each affirmation be lived fully; 'busy' not be a reason to not do anything and your hearts spring forth into eternity; healing life on this planet and humans passed into other dimensions!" Most importantly, may you always honor all that you are and that is within you.

Giagia Pagona's words echo daily in my ears: the importance of being true to yourself, no matter what another thinks of you. Most importantly, MAY YOU ALWAYS HONOR ALL THAT YOU ARE AND THAT IS WITHIN YOU.

SOUL INGREDIENTS

BIBLIOGRAPHY

Allen, James. *As A Man Thinketh*. Peter Pauper Press, New York

Baggott, Andy. *Blissology: The Art and Science of Happiness,* Llewellyn Publications, 2011

Bartlett, Richard, DC, ND. *The Physics of Miracles: tapping into the field of consciousness potential*. Atria Books/Beyond Words Publishing, 2009

Batmanghelidj, F. MD. *Obesity, Cancer, Depression*. Global Health Solutions, Falls Church, VA 2005

Braden, Gregg. *Fractal Time: The Secret of 2012 and a New World Age*. Hay House, 2009

Carroll, Lee. *The Twelve Layers of DNA (An Esoteric Study of the Mastery Within)* Kryon Book 12. Platinum Publishing House, 2010

Cherniske, Stephen, M.S., *Caffeine Blues*. Warner Books, 1998

Chia, Mantak. *Healing Love through the Tao*. Destiny Books, 2005

Chopra, Deepak. *The Path to Love*. Harmony Books, 1995

Covey, Stephen R. *The 7 Habits of Highly Effective People*. Simon and Schuster, 1990

Dass, Ram and Bush, Mirabai. *Compassion In Action: Setting Out on the Path of Service*. Bell Tower, 1992

Demartini, John F. *The Breakthrough Experience: a revolutionary new approach to personal transformation*. Hay House, 2002

Eker, Harv T. *Secrets of the Millionaire Mind: Mastering the Inner Game of Wealth*. Harper Collins, 2005

Esko, Wendy. *Introducing Macrobiotic Cooking*. Japan Publications Inc. 1978

Ewald, Buchman Ellen. *Recipes for a Small Planet*. Ballantine Books, New York, 1973

Feldhahn, Shaunti. *For women only*. Multnomah Publishers, Sisters, Oregon 2004

Frankl, Victor E. *Man's Search for Meaning*. Simon and Schuster. New York, 1959

Gagné, Steve. *Food Energetics: the spiritual, emotional and nutritional power of what we eat*. Healing Arts Press, 1990, 2006, 2008

Gawain, Shakti. *The Four Levels of Healing*. Nataraj Publishing, 1997

Gribbin, John. *In Search of Schrodinger's Cat*. Bantam Books, Toronto, 1984.

Gyurme Dorje, translator. *Meditations on Living, Dying and Loss: Ancient Knowledge for a Modern World from the First Complete Translation of the Tibetan Book of the Dead*. Viking, 2005

Hanh, Thich Nhat. *Peace is Every Step*. Bantam Books, 1991

Heiss, Mary Lou and Heiss, Robert J. *The Story of Tea: A Cultural History and Drinking Guide*. Ten Speed Press, 2007

Higley, Connie and Alan Higley. *Reference Guide for Essential Oils. Abundant Health*, Spanish Fork, UT, 2010

Hill, Napoleon. Rev. and expanded by Pell, Arthur R. *Think and Grow Rich*. Penguin Group, 2003, 2005

Holliwell, Raymond, Dr. *Working with The Law*. Life Success Productions 2007, 2004, 1964

Icke, David. *Human Race Get Off Your Knees, The Lion Sleeps No More*. David Icke Books, 2010

Javane, Faith and Bunker, Dusty. *Numerology and The Divine Triangle*. Schiffer Publishing, 1979

Jensen, Bernard D.C. *Vital Foods for Total Health*. American Offset Printers, 1984

Jordan, Michael. *I Can't Accept Not Trying: Michael Jordan on The Pursuit of Excellence*. Harper San Francisco, 1994

Kaptchuk, Ted J. *The Web That Has No Weaver*. Contemporary Books, 2000

Keating, Kathleen. *The Hug Therapy Book*. Hazelden Foundation, 1983

Lipton, Bruce H. and Bhaerman, Steve. *Spontaneous Evolution: our positive future (and a way to get there from here)*. Hay House, 2009

Maciocia, Giovanni. *The Foundations of Chinese Medicine*. Churchill Livingstone, 1989

Maddock-Dewhurst, Olivea. *The book of sound therapy: heal yourself with music and voice*. Simon and Schuster, 1993

Maltz, Maxwell, M.D. F.I.C.S. *The New Psycho-Cybernetics*. Prentice Hall Press, 2001

Mah, Adeline Yen. *Watching the Tree: A Chinese Daughter Reflects on Happiness, Tradition and Spiritual Wisdom*. Broadway Books, New York, 2001

Mandino, Og. *The Greatest Miracle in The World*. Random House, 1983

McBride-Campbell, Natasha, MD. *Gut and Psychology Syndrome*. Medinform Publishing, 2010

McBride-Campbell, Natasha, MD. *Put Your Heart in Your Mouth*. Medinform Publishing, 2007

McColl, Peggy. *Your Destiny Switch: Master Your Key Emotions and Attract the Life of Your Dreams*. Hay House, 2007

Melngailis, Sarma. *Living Raw Food: get the glow with more recipes from Pure Food and Wine.* William Morrow, 2009

Osho. *Emotional Wellness: Transforming fear, anger and jealousy into creative energy.* Harmony Books, New York, 2007

Pellegrino-Estrich, Robert. *The Power to Heal.* Brazil, 2008

Praagh, James Van. *Heaven and Earth.* Pocket Books, 2001

Proctor, Bob. *You Were Born Rich.* Life Success Productions, 1984, 1997, 2002

Provine, Robert R. Laughter: *A Scientific Investigation.* Viking Penguin Books, 2000

Rosenthal, Joshua. *Integrative Nutrition.* Integrative Nutrition Publishing, 2008

Sawyer, Karen. *The Dangerous Man.* O Books, 2010

Simpkins, Annellen M. and Simpkins Alexander C., *Zen Around the World,* Tuttle Publishing, 1997

Sirota, Golda. *Love Food.* Living Loving Learning Center, 1984

Somé, Sobonfu E. *Falling Out of Grace.* North Bay Books, California, 2003

Svirinskaya, Alla. *Energy Secrets. The Ultimate Well-Being Plan.* Hay House, 2005

Tolle, Eckhart. *The Power of Now: A Guide to Spiritual Enlightenment.* New World Library, 1999

Tzu, Lao translated by Wu, John C.H. *Tao Te Ching.* Shambala, Boston and London, 1989

Walsch, Neale Donald. *Conversations With God*, Book 1. G.P. Putnam's Sons, 1995

Walsch, Neale Donald. *Conversations With God, Book 2.* Hampton Roads Publishing Company, Inc. 1997, 2012

Walsch, Neale Donald. *Conversations With God, Book 3.* Hampton Roads Publishing Company, Inc. 1997, 2012

Wilber, Ken. *The Integral Vision: A Very Short Introduction to the Revolutionary Integral Approach to Life, God, the Universe and Everything.* Shambhala, Boston and London, 2007

Wilcock, David. *The Source Field Investigations: The Hidden Science Behind the 2012 Prophecies.* Plume, 2012

Wigmore, Ann. *Recipes for Longer Life.* Rising Sun Publications,1978

Wigmore, Ann. *The Wheatgrass Book. How to Grow and Use Wheatgrass to Maximize Your Health and Vitality.* Avery Trade, 1985

Zi, Nancy. *The Art of Breathing.* Bantam Books, 1986

SOUL INGREDIENTS

WEBSITES
(Note: Websites may have changed/been deleted since book was written)

ACUPRESSURE:
www.acupressure.com

ACUPUNCTURE:
www.aaom.org
www.medicalacupuncture.org
www.nesa.org
www.nccaom.org
www.tai.edu

A HEALER'S GUIDE TO NATURAL HEALTH:
www.watercure.com

ALEXANDER TECHNIQUE:
www.alexandertech.com

ALTERNATIVE RESEARCH COMMUNITY CONVENTIONS (ARC):
www.ArcConvention.org

AROMATHERAPY:
www.naha.org
www.pacificinstituteofaromatherapy.com

ARVIGO TECHNIQUES OF MAYA ABDOMINAL THERAPY™:
www.arvigotherapy.com

ASSOCIATION FOR RESEARCH & ENLIGHTENMENT, INC. (A.R.E)
www.EdgarCayce.org

ASTROLOGY:
http://www.astrologycom.com/index.html

SOUL INGREDIENTS

AYURVEDA:
www.ayurveda.com

CENTERS FOR ADVANCED HEALING:
www.centerforadvancedmedicine.com

CHELATION THERAPY:
www.abct.info
www.acam.org

CHIOS ENERGY HEALING:
http://www.chioshealing.com

CHIROPRACTIC:
www.amerchiro.org
www.chiropractic.org
www.worldchiropracticalliance.org

COLON THERAPY/HYDROTHERAPY:
www.i-act.org

RUPERT DAVIS, visionary artist:
www.newearthphotography.com

DIAMOND ALIGNMENT:
http://www.divinediamondhealing.com/index.php

ORIBEL DIVINE, animal & interspecies communicator:
www.oribeldivine.com

ESSENTIAL OILS:
www.youngliving.com

FELDENKRAIS:
www.feldenkrais.com

PAGONA

GAPS:
www.gaps.me
www.scdiet.org
www.pagona.com

GLOBAL CONSCIOUSNESS PROJECT:
www.boundaryinstitute.org/randomness.htm

HAKOMI INSTITUTE:
www.hakomiinstitute.com

HELLERWORK:
www.hellerwork.com

HENDRICKS INSTITUTE:
www.hendricks.com

HUNGRY FOR CHANGE DOCUMENTARY:
www.hungryforchangetv.com

KINESIOLOGY:
http://www.quantumtouch.com
www.icak.com
www.uskinesiologyinstitute.com

LEE HARRIS:
www.leeharrisenergy.com

NATUROPATHIC:
www.hanp.net

OSTEOPATHIC MEDICINE:
www.academyofosteopathic.org
www.cranialacademy.com
www.holisticmedicine.org

PSYCHO-CYBERNETICS:
www.psycho-cybernetics.com

REFLEXOLOGY:
www.reflexology-usa.org

REIKI:
www.reiki.org

ROLFING:
www.rolf.org

ROSEN METHOD:
www.rosenmethod.org

THE WAY TO BALANCE (Sue and Aaron Singleton):
www.thewaytobalance.com

TONING:
http://www.lemurianchoir.com/the-pineal-tones

TOTAL INTEGRATION THERAPY:
www.livingfreedom.net
www.touch4healing.com

TRAGER APPROACH:
www.trager.com

UNIVERSAL HEALING CENTER:
www.universal-tao.com

VANISHING OF THE BEES:
www.vanishingbees.com

SOUL INGREDIENTS

VIPASSANA MEDITATION:
www.dharma.org

WESTON PRICE FOUNDATION:
www.westonaprice.org

SOUL INGREDIENTS